Pocket Atlas of
Cross-Sectional
Anatomy
Volume 2

Pocket Atlas of Cross-Sectional Anatomy

Computed Tomography and Magnetic Resonance Imaging

Volume 2:

Thorax, Abdomen, and Pelvis

Torsten B. Möller and Emil Reif

Translated by Clifford Bergman

450 Illustrations

1994
Georg Thieme Verlag Stuttgart · New York
Thieme Medical Publishers, Inc. New York

Dr. Torsten B. Möller
Dr. Emil Reif
Am Caritas-Krankenhaus
66763 Dillingen/Saar
Germany

Clifford Bergman, M.D.
Eglingerstr. 10
82544 Moosham
Germany

Cover design by
D. Loenicker, Stuttgart

© 1994 Georg Thieme Verlag,
Rüdigerstraße 14, 70469 Stuttgart
Germany
Thieme Medical Publishers, Inc., 381 Park Avenue South, New York, N.Y. 10016

Typesetting by Fotosatz Froitzheim,
53113 Bonn, set on MS-DOS PC
with Aldus Freehand
Printed in Germany by Karl Grammlich,
72124 Pliezhausen

ISBN 3-13-125601-X (GTV, Stuttgart)
ISBN 0-86577-511-7 (TMP, New York)

Library of Congress
Cataloging-in-Publication Data

Möller, Torsten B.
[Taschenatlas der Schnittbildanatomie. English]
Pocket atlas of cross-sectional anatomy : computed tomography and magnetic resonance imaging / Torsten Möller, Emil Reif : translated by Clifford Bergman.
p. cm.
Includes bibliographical references and index.
Contents: v. 1. Head, neck, spine, and joints – v. 2. Thorax, abdomen, and pelvis.
1. Human anatomy-Atlases. 2. Tomography-Atlases. 3. Magnetic resonance imaging-Atlases. I. Reif, Emil. II. Title.
[DNLM. 1. Anatomy, Regional-atlases.
2. Tomography, X-Ray-Computed-Atlases.
3. Magnetic Resonance Imaging-atlases.
QS 17 M726t 1994a]
QM25.M55513 1994 611'.9'0222-dc20 DNLM/
DLC

Dedicated to the American part of our roots
the
Riegner Family, Michigan
and
Ronge Family, Connecticut

Preface

This atlas presents the basic anatomy needed to interpret CT and MR images.

Diagnosis with cross-sectional images requires an adaption in thinking, even among experienced clinicians, to this specific form of anatomy. For this reason, this atlas presents both of the currently most important cross-sectional imaging technologies.

One of the reasons these techniques play such a significant role today is that they afford a very high resolution. Therefore it was important to us that this book remain compact and concise, in spite of its comprehensiveness in including all anatomic structures. The four-color illustrations were essential to this success.

The two volumes are each halves of a whole work, which is organized along strict lines: each image is accompanied by a color-coded diagram, which we drew ourselves to avoid inaccuracies. Schematic drawings showing the level of the cross section completes the spectrum of information necessary to interpret the image.

All images were done on patients or volunteers. For their ongoing support during the creation of this book, we thank our radiologic technicians and assistants, especially Michalea Knittel, Pia Saar, Gisela Wagner, Monjuri Paul, and Andrea Britz. The manuscript was typed by Helga Brettschneider and Gabi Müller. Special thanks to Dr. Markus Bach, Dr. Patrick Rosar, and especially Dr. Beate Hilpert for reading the manuscript and making helpful suggestions.

Dillingen, December 1993   Torsten B. Möller and Emil Reif

Table of Contents

Thorax

Abdomen

Pelvis

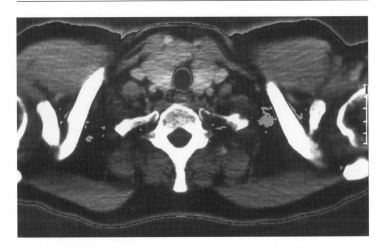

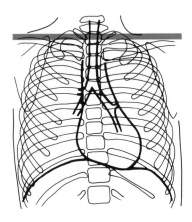

1 Pectoralis minor muscle
2 Posterior scalene muscle
3 Medial scalene muscle
4 Anterior scalene muscle
5 Sternohyoid muscle
6 Sternocleidomastoid muscle
7 Thyroid gland
8 Esophagus
9 Trachea
10 External jugular vein
11 Longus colli muscle
12 Common carotid artery
13 Internal jugular vein
14 Apex of lung
15 Pectoralis major muscle
16 Subscapularis muscle
17 Axillary vein
18 Axillary artery
19 Head of humerus

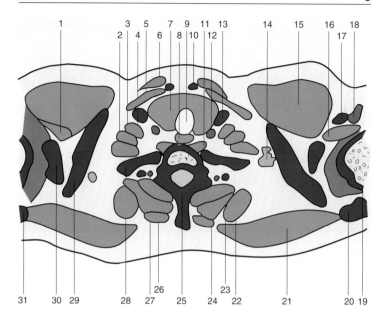

20 Acromion
21 Trapezius muscle
22 Levator scapulae muscle
23 Semispinalis capitis muscle
24 Splenius capitis muscle
25 Thoracic vertebra 1
26 Lesser rhomboid muscle
27 Deep cervical artery and vein
28 Rib 1
29 Clavicle
30 Coracoid process
31 Acromion
32 Supraclavicular lymph nodes
33 Jugular lymph nodes
34 Thyroid lymph nodes
35 Paratracheal lymph nodes
36 Anterior cervical lymph nodes
37 Retropharyngeal lymph nodes

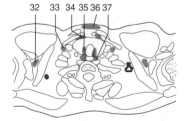

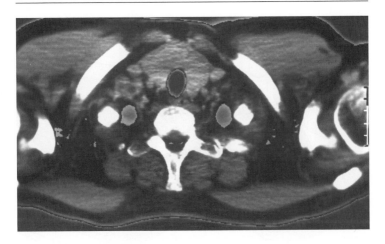

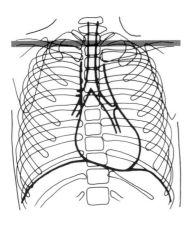

1 Clavicle
2 Anterior and medial scalene muscles
3 Internal jugular vein
4 Common carotid artery
5 Longus colli muscle
6 Trachea
7 Esophagus
8 External jugular vein
9 Thyroid gland
10 Sternocleidomastoid muscle
11 Apex of lung
12 Anterior scalene muscle
13 Rib 1
14 Medial scalene muscle
15 Pectoralis major muscle
16 Pectoralis minor muscle
17 Axillary artery and vein
18 Deltoid muscle
19 Spine of scapula

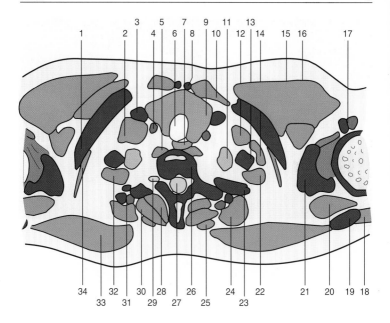

20 Supraspinatus muscle
21 Neck of scapula
22 Posterior scalene muscle
23 Rib 1
24 Levator scapulae muscle
25 Rhomboid muscle
26 Thoracic vertebra 2
27 Spinal canal, dural sac
28 Semispinalis capitis muscle
29 Spinalis muscle 1
30 Splenius capitis muscle
31 Deep cervical artery and vein
32 Posterior scalene muscle
33 Trapezius muscle
34 Omohyoid muscle
35 Thyroid lymph nodes
36 Retropharyngeal lymph nodes
37 Anterior cervical lymph nodes
38 Paratracheal lymph nodes

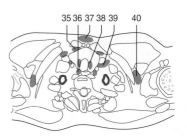

39 Jugular lymph nodes
40 Supraclavicular lymph nodes

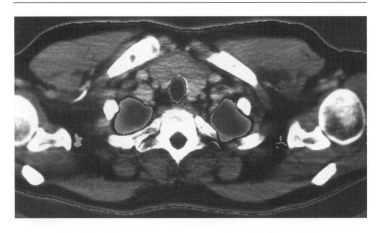

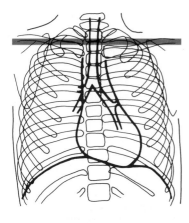

1 Subclavian artery
2 Pectoralis minor muscle
3 Pectoralis major muscle
4 Rib 1
5 Deltoid muscle
6 Subclavian artery
7 Common carotid artery
8 Longus colli muscle
9 Sternocleidomastoid muscle
10 Trachea
11 Esophagus
12 External jugular vein
13 Thyroid gland
14 Sternohyoid and sternothyroid muscles
15 Internal jugular vein
16 Clavicle, sternal extremity
17 Subclavius muscle
18 Subscapularis muscle
19 Subclavian vein

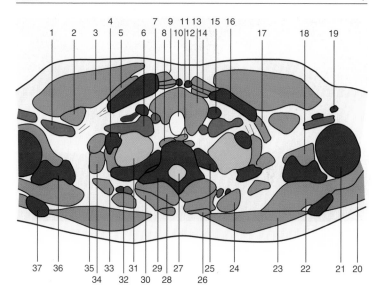

20 M. deltoideus
21 Head of humerus
22 Supraspinatus muscle
23 Trapezius muscle
24 Levator scapulae muscle
25 Head of rib 2
26 Rhomboid muscle
27 Spinal canal
28 Semispinalis capitis muscle
29 Transverse process of thoracic
   vertebra 2
30 Splenius capitis muscle
31 Apex of lung
32 Deep cervical artery and vein
33 Posterior scalene muscle
34 Medial scalene muscle
35 Anterior scalene muscle
36 Neck of scapula

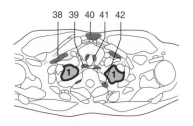

37 Spine of scapula
38 Deep axillary lymph nodes
39 Retropharyngeal and prevertebral
   lymph nodes
40 Anterior cervical lymph nodes
41 Paratracheal lymph nodes
42 Posterior intercostal lymph nodes

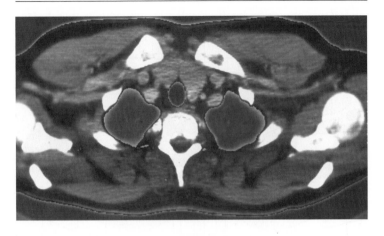

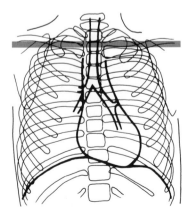

1 Pectoralis minor muscle
2 Pectoralis major muscle
3 Clavicle, sternal extremity
4 Sternocleidomastoid muscle
5 Sternohyoid and sternothyroid muscles
6 Trachea
7 Esophagus
8 Thyroid gland
9 Common carotid artery
10 Subclavian artery
11 Internal jugular vein
12 Left subclavian vein
13 Left subclavian artery
14 Deltoid muscle
15 Infraspinatus muscle
16 Head of humerus
17 Neck of scapula
18 Subscapularis muscle
19 Supraspinatus muscle

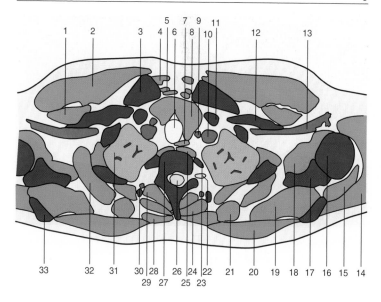

20 Trapezius muscle
21 Levator scapulae muscle
22 Nerve root
23 Head of rib
24 Splenius capitis muscle
25 Longus colli muscle
26 Dural sac
27 Thoracic vertebra 2
28 Rhomboid muscle
29 Semispinalis capitis muscle
30 Deep cervical artery and vein
31 Apex of lung
32 Serratus anterior muscle
33 Spine of scapula
34 Interpectoral lymph nodes
35 Posterior intercostal lymph nodes
36 Paratracheal lymph nodes
37 Anterior cervical lymph nodes

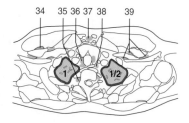

38 Retropharyngeal and prevertebral
   lymph nodes
39 Deep axillary lymph nodes

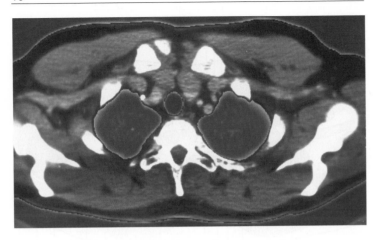

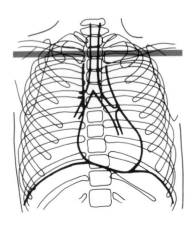

1 Pectoralis minor muscle
2 Pectoralis major muscle
3 Subclavius muscle
4 Clavicle, sternal extremity
5 Brachiocephalic trunk
6 Sternum
7 Sternothyroid and sternohyoid
   muscles
8 Trachea
9 Esophagus
10 Sternocleidomastoid muscle
11 Thyroid gland
12 Common carotid artery
13 Subclavian artery
14 Subclavian vein
15 Subscapularis muscle
16 Head of humerus
17 Teres major muscle
18 Infraspinatus muscle

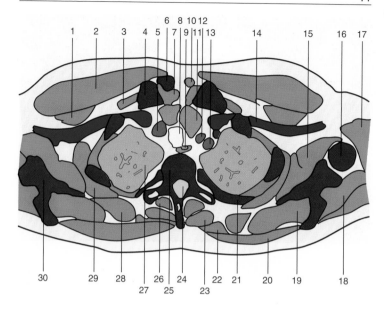

19 Supraspinatus muscle
20 Trapezius muscle
21 Rib 3
22 Rhomboid muscle
23 Splenius capitis muscle
24 Dural sac
25 Thoracic vertebra 3
26 Semispinalis capitis muscle
27 Right lung
28 Levator scapulae muscle
29 Serratus anterior muscle
30 Neck of scapula
31 Superficial axillary lymph nodes
32 Interpectoral lymph nodes
33 Deep axillary lymph nodes
34 Paratracheal lymph nodes
35 Prevertebral lymph nodes
36 Retropharyngeal lymph nodes
37 Anterior mediastinal lymph nodes

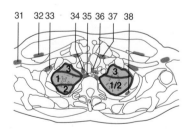

38 Intercostal lymph nodes

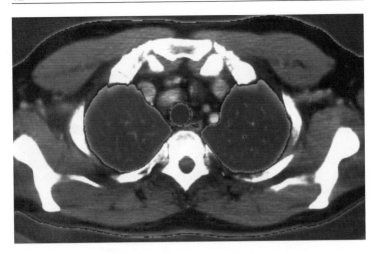

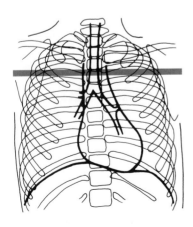

1 Axillary artery
2 Pectoralis major muscle
3 Pectoralis minor muscle
4 Rib 1
5 Clavicle
6 Brachiocephalic trunk
7 Inferior thyroid artery and vein
8 Sternohyoid and sternothyroid
   muscles
9 Trachea
10 Manubrium of sternum
11 Esophagus
12 Thyroid gland
13 Common carotid artery
14 Subclavian artery
15 Brachiocephalic vein
16 Subclavian vein
17 Teres major muscle
18 Teres minor muscle

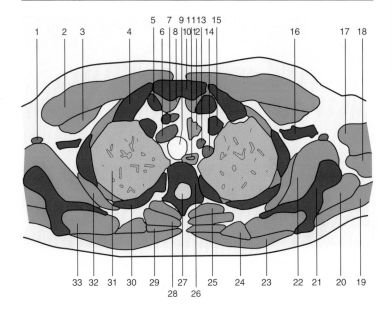

19 Deltoid muscle
20 Infraspinatus muscle
21 Scapula
22 Subscapularis muscle
23 Trapezius muscle
24 Levator scapulae muscle
25 Semispinalis capitis muscle
26 Thoracic vertebra 3
27 Spinal canal
28 Splenius capitis muscle
29 Rhomboid muscle
30 Rib 3
31 Right lung
32 Serratus anterior muscle
33 Supraspinatus muscle
34 Deep axillary lymph nodes
35 Intercostal lymph nodes
36 Paratracheal lymph nodes
37 Prevertebral lymph nodes

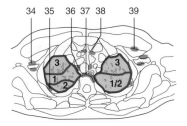

38 Anterior mediastinal lymph nodes
39 Interpectoral lymph nodes

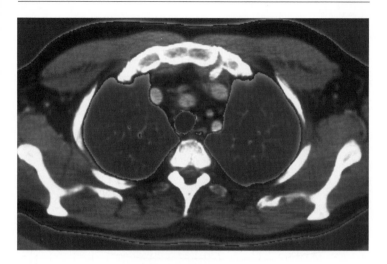

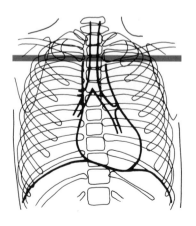

1 Thoracodorsal artery
2 Pectoralis minor muscle
3 Pectoralis major muscle
4 Left lung
5 Brachiocephalic vein
6 Sternohyoid and sternothyroid
  muscles
7 Trachea
8 Inferior thyroid vein
9 Brachiocephalic trunk
10 Sternum
11 Esophagus
12 Common carotid artery
13 Clavicle
14 Left lung
15 Subscapularis muscle
16 Triceps muscle (long head)
17 Teres major muscle
18 Deltoid muscle

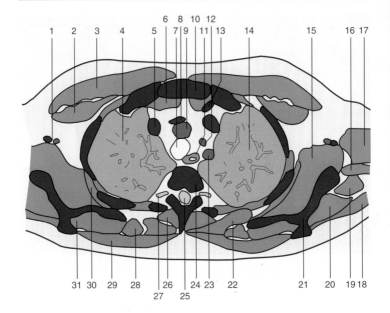

19 Teres minor muscle
20 Supraspinatus muscle
21 Scapula
22 Rhomboid muscle
23 Subclavian artery
24 Thoracic vertebra 4
25 Dural sac
26 Erector spinae muscle
27 Spinal nerve root
28 Levator scapulae muscle
29 Trapezius muscle
30 Serratus anterior muscle
31 Supraspinatus muscle
32 Superficial axillary lymph nodes
33 Anterior mediastinal lymph nodes
34 Prevertebral lymph nodes
35 Paratracheal lymph nodes
36 Intercostal lymph nodes
37 Interpectoral lymph nodes

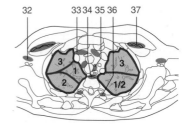

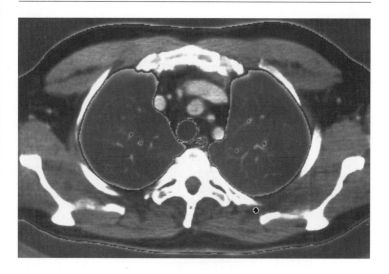

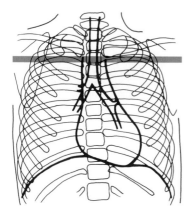

1 Thoracodorsal artery
2 Thoracodorsal vein
3 Pectoralis minor muscle
4 Pectoralis major muscle
5 Right lung
6 Right brachiocephalic vein
7 Sternum
8 Inferior thyroid vein
9 Trachea
10 Brachiocephalic trunk
11 Left brachiocephalic vein
12 Common carotid artery
13 Subclavian artery
14 Left lung
15 Subscapularis muscle
16 Latissimus dorsi muscle
17 Teres major muscle
18 Deltoid muscle
19 Infraspinatus muscle

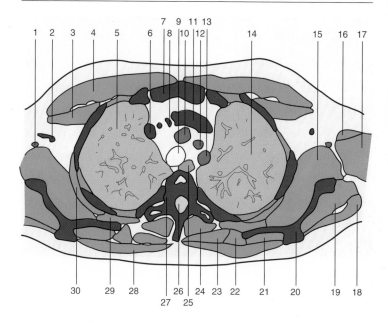

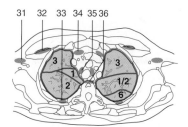

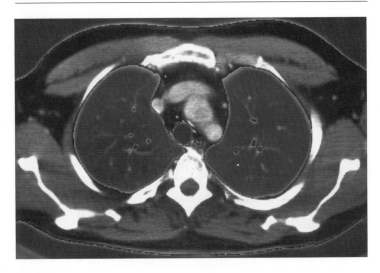

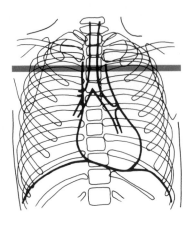

 1 Thoracodorsal artery
 2 Pectoralis minor muscle
 3 Pectoralis major muscle
 4 Right lung
 5 Internal thoracic artery
 6 Right brachiocephalic vein
 7 Sternum
 8 Trachea
 9 Left brachiocephalic vein
10 Esophagus
11 Brachiocephalic trunk
12 Subclavian artery
13 Internal thoracic vein
14 Left lung
15 Thoracodorsal vein
16 Latissimus dorsi muscle
17 Teres major muscle
18 Deltoid muscle
19 Circumflex scapular artery

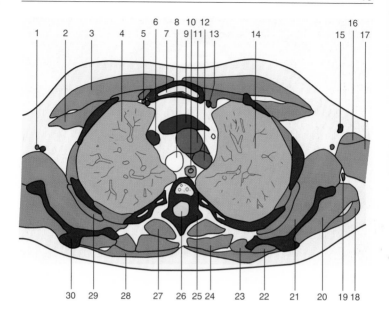

20 Infraspinatus muscle
21 Subscapularis muscle
22 Supraspinatus muscle
23 Levator scapulae muscle
24 Rhomboid muscle
25 Thoracic vertebra 5
26 Spinal canal
27 Erector spinae muscle
28 Trapezius muscle
29 Serratus anterior muscle
30 Scapula
31 Superficial axillary lymph nodes
32 Interpectoral lymph nodes
33 Intercostal lymph nodes
34 Paratracheal lymph nodes
35 Prevertebral lymph nodes
36 Anterior mediastinal lymph nodes

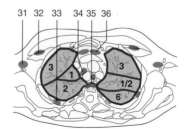

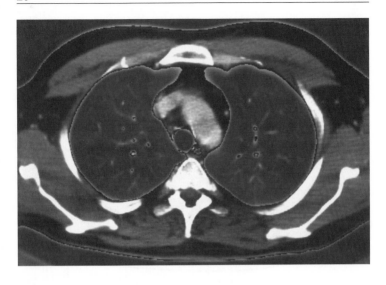

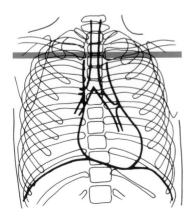

1 Thoracodorsal artery
2 Pectoralis minor muscle
3 Pectoralis major muscle
4 Right lung
5 Superior vena cava
6 Trachea
7 Sternum
8 Esophagus
9 Aortic arch
10 Internal thoracic artery and vein
11 Left lung
12 Thoracodorsal vein
13 Circumflex scapular artery
14 Latissimus dorsi muscle
15 Teres major muscle
16 Teres minor muscle
17 Deltoid muscle
18 Serratus anterior muscle
19 Levator scapulae muscle

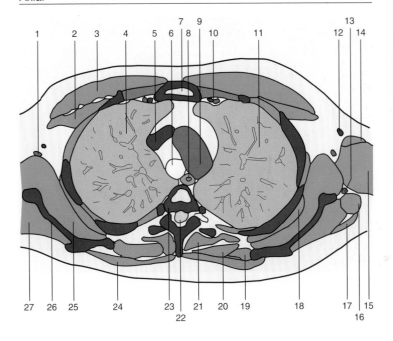

20 Rhomboid muscle
21 Erector spinae muscle
22 Dural sac
23 Thoracic vertebra 5
24 Trapezius muscle
25 Subscapularis muscle
26 Scapula
27 Infraspinatus muscle
28 Superficial axillary lymph nodes
29 Parasternal lymph nodes
30 Paratracheal lymph nodes
31 Prevertebral lymph nodes
32 Anterior mediastinal lymph nodes
33 Intercostal lymph nodes
34 Interpectoral lymph nodes

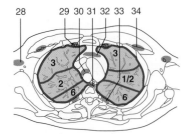

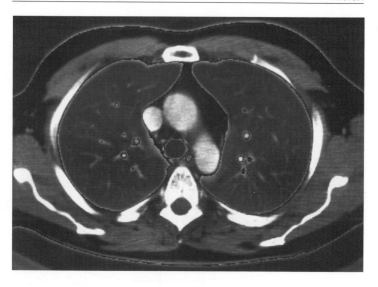

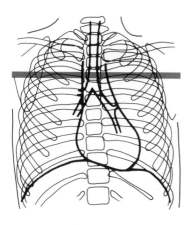

1 Thoracodorsal artery and vein
2 Pectoralis minor muscle
3 Pectoralis major muscle
4 Right lung
5 Superior vena cava
6 Sternum
7 Trachea
8 Esophagus
9 Aortic arch
10 Left lung
11 Subscapularis muscle
12 Teres major muscle
13 Latissimus dorsi muscle
14 Teres minor muscle
15 Deltoid muscle
16 Infraspinatus muscle
17 Erector spinae muscle
18 Spinal canal
19 Thoracic vertebra 6

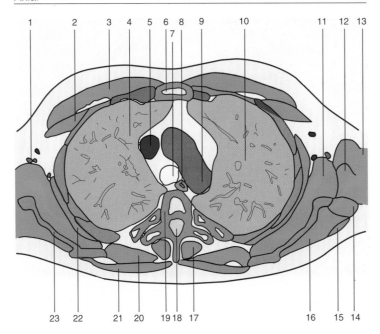

20 Rhomboid muscle
21 Trapezius muscle
22 Serratus anterior muscle
23 Scapula
24 Superficial axillary lymph nodes
25 Interpectoral lymph nodes
26 Parasternal lymph nodes
27 Paratracheal lymph nodes
28 Prevertebral lymph nodes
29 Anterior mediastinal lymph nodes
30 Intercostal lymph nodes

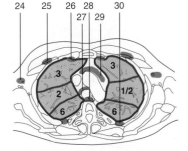

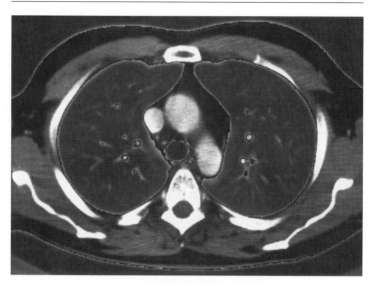

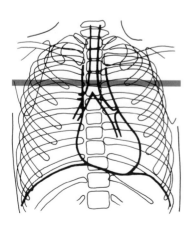

1 Thoracodorsal artery and vein
2 Pectoralis minor muscle
3 Pectoralis major muscle
4 Right lung
5 Superior vena cava
6 Sternum
7 Trachea
8 Aortic arch
9 Esophagus
10 Descending aorta
11 Internal thoracic artery and vein
12 Left lung
13 Serratus anterior muscle
14 Latissimus dorsi muscle
15 Teres major muscle
16 Teres minor muscle
17 Infraspinatus muscle
18 Subscapularis muscle
19 Trapezius muscle

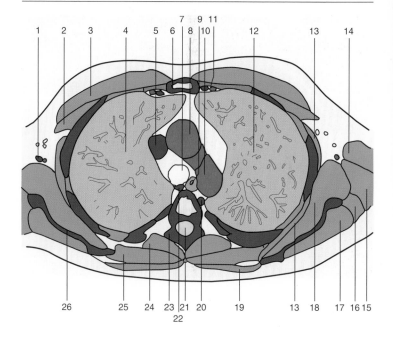

20 Hemiazygos vein
21 Spinal canal
22 Azygos vein
23 Thoracic vertebra 6
24 Erector spinae muscle
25 Rhomboid muscle
26 Scapula
27 Superficial axillary lymph nodes
28 Interpectoral lymph nodes
29 Intercostal lymph nodes
30 Parasternal lymph nodes
31 Paratracheal lymph nodes
32 Prevertebral lymph nodes
33 Anterior mediastinal lymph nodes

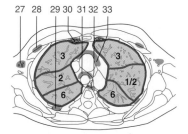

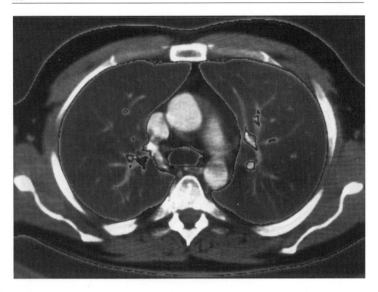

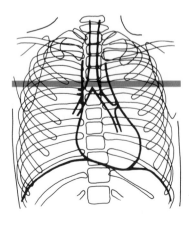

1 Serratus anterior muscle
2 Pectoralis minor muscle
3 Pectoralis major muscle
4 Right pulmonary artery
5 Superior vena cava
6 Sternum
7 Trachea (bifurcation)
8 Ascending aorta
9 Descending aorta
10 Internal thoracic artery and vein
11 Left pulmonary artery
12 Thoracodorsal artery and vein
13 Latissimus dorsi muscle
14 Teres major muscle
15 Teres minor muscle
16 Rhomboid muscle
17 Thoracic vertebra 6
18 Hemiazygos vein
19 Esophagus

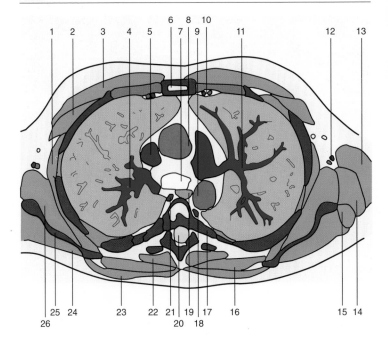

20 Dural sac
21 Azygos vein
22 Erector spinae muscle
23 Trapezius muscle
24 Infraspinatus muscle
25 Scapula
26 Subscapularis muscle
27 Paramammary lymph nodes
28 Intercostal lymph nodes
29 Anterior mediastinal lymph nodes
30 Paratracheal lymph nodes
31 Prevertebral lymph nodes
32 Parasternal lymph nodes
33 Juxtaesophageal lymph nodes

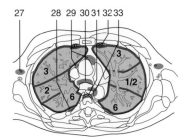

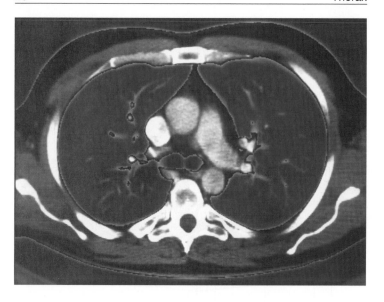

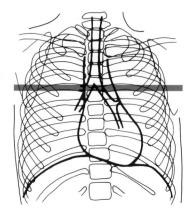

1 Pectoralis minor muscle
2 Pectoralis major muscle
3 Right pulmonary artery
4 Right superior lobar bronchus
5 Superior vena cava
6 Right main stem bronchus
7 Sternum
8 Descending aorta
9 Left main stem bronchus
10 Hemiazygos vein
11 Internal thoracic artery and vein
12 Left pulmonary artery
13 Left superior lobar bronchus
14 Thoracodorsal artery and vein
15 Teres major muscle
16 Latissimus dorsi muscle
17 Rhomboid muscle
18 Erector spinae muscle
19 Descending aorta

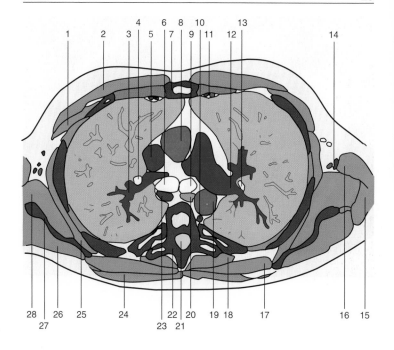

28 | 26 | 25 | 24 | 22 | 20 | 19 | 18 | 17 | 16 | 15
27 | 23 | 21 | 14

20 Esophagus
21 Spinal canal
22 Thoracic vertebra 7
23 Azygos vein
24 Trapezius muscle
25 Serratus anterior muscle
26 Infraspinatus muscle
27 Scapula
28 Subscapularis muscle
29 Paramammary lymph nodes
30 Intercostal lymph nodes
31 Tracheobronchial lymph nodes
32 Juxtaesophageal lymph nodes
33 Parasternal lymph nodes
34 Anterior mediastinal lymph nodes

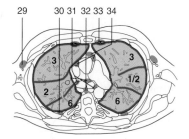

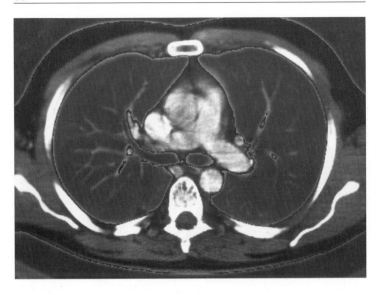

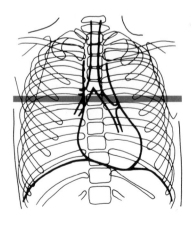

1 Thoracodorsal artery and vein
2 Pectoralis minor muscle
3 Pectoralis major muscle
4 Right pulmonary vein
5 Right pulmonary artery
6 Superior vena cava
7 Ascending aorta
8 Sternum
9 Right atrial appendage
10 Left main stem bronchus
11 Right ventricle
12 Internal thoracic artery and vein
13 Pulmonary trunk
14 Left pulmonary artery
15 Left superior lobar bronchus
16 Subscapularis muscle
17 Latissimus dorsi muscle
18 Teres major muscle
19 Infraspinatus muscle

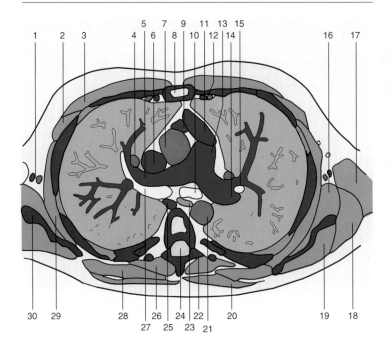

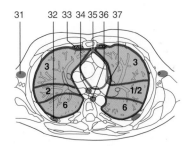

20 Trapezius muscle
21 Descending aorta
22 Thoracic vertebra 7
23 Esophagus
24 Spinal canal
25 Azygos vein
26 Erector spinae muscle
27 Right main stem bronchus
28 Rhomboid muscle
29 Serratus anterior muscle
30 Scapula
31 Paramammary lymph nodes
32 Intercostal lymph nodes
33 Parasternal lymph nodes
34 Inferior tracheobronchial lymph nodes
35 Anterior mediastinal lymph nodes
36 Juxtaesophageal lymph nodes
37 Bronchopulmonary lymph nodes

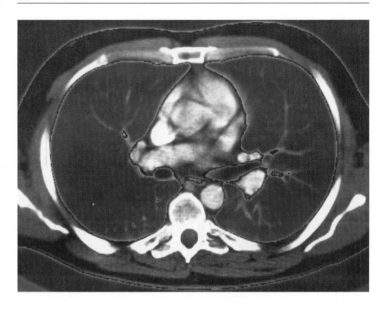

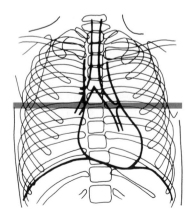

1 Thoracodorsal artery and vein
2 Pectoralis minor muscle
3 Pectoralis major muscle
4 Superior vena cava
5 Right inferior lobar bronchus
6 Right atrium
7 Right pulmonary vein
8 Sternum
9 Ascending aorta
10 Descending aorta
11 Internal thoracic artery and vein
12 Right ventricle
13 Pulmonary trunk
14 Subscapularis muscle
15 Latissimus dorsi muscle
16 Teres major muscle
17 Infraspinatus muscle
18 Left pulmonary artery
19 Left pulmonary vein

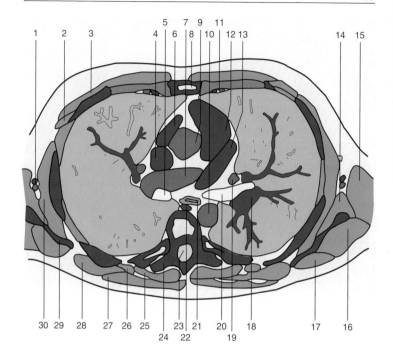

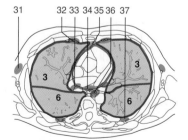

20 Left main stem bronchus
21 Esophagus
22 Azygos vein
23 Spinal canal
24 Thoracic vertebra 7
25 Erector spinae muscle
26 Serratus anterior muscle
27 Trapezius muscle
28 Rhomboid muscle
29 Scapula
30 Serratus anterior muscle
31 Paramammary lymph nodes
32 Parasternal lymph nodes
33 Bronchopulmonary lymph nodes
34 Inferior tracheobronchial lymph nodes
35 Anterior mediastinal lymph nodes
36 Juxtaesophageal lymph nodes
37 Intercostal lymph nodes

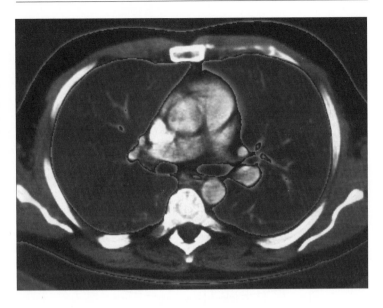

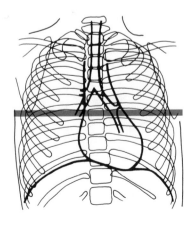

1 Thoracodorsal artery and vein
2 Pectoralis minor muscle
3 Pectoralis major muscle
4 Right pulmonary vein
5 Internal thoracic artery and vein
6 Superior vena cava
7 Right atrium
8 Right pulmonary vein
9 Sternum
10 Ascending aorta
11 Right ventricle
12 Left pulmonary vein
13 Left atrial appendage
14 Left pulmonary vein
15 Left pulmonary vein
16 Serratus anterior muscle
17 Latissimus dorsi muscle
18 Teres major muscle
19 Subscapularis muscle

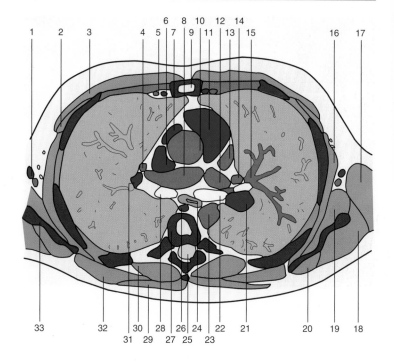

20 Infraspinatus muscle
21 Left pulmonary artery
22 Left main stem bronchus
23 Descending aorta
24 Esophagus
25 Spinal canal
26 Azygos vein
27 Thoracic vertebra 7
28 Right inferior lobar bronchus
29 Trapezius muscle
30 Erector spinae muscle
31 Right pulmonary artery
32 Rhomboid muscle
33 Scapula
34 Paramammary lymph nodes
35 Intercostal lymph nodes
36 Bronchopulmonary lymph nodes
37 Parasternal lymph nodes
38 Inferior tracheobronchial lymph nodes

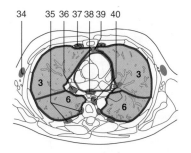

39 Inferior prepericardial lymph nodes
40 Juxtaesophageal lymph nodes

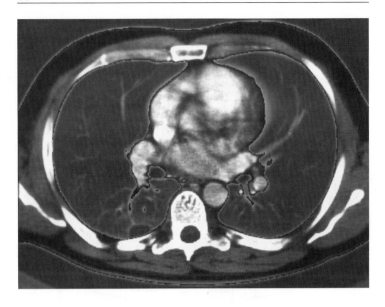

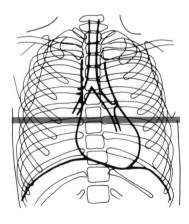

1 Thoracodorsal artery and vein
2 Serratus anterior muscle
3 Pectoralis major muscle
4 Right pulmonary vein
5 Right inferior lobar bronchus
6 Superior vena cava
7 Right atrium
8 Esophagus
9 Sternum
10 Descending aorta
11 Left atrium
12 Internal thoracic artery and vein
13 Right ventricle
14 Left atrial appendage
15 Left pulmonary vein
16 Subscapularis muscle
17 Latissimus dorsi muscle
18 Teres major muscle
19 Infraspinatus muscle

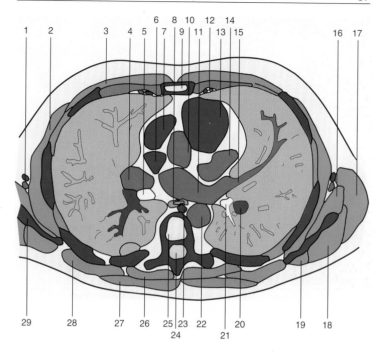

20 Left pulmonary artery
21 Left inferior lobar bronchus
22 Descending aorta
23 Azygos vein
24 Spinal canal
25 Thoracic vertebra 8
26 Erector spinae muscle
27 Trapezius muscle
28 Rhomboid muscle
29 Scapula
30 Paramammary lymph nodes
31 Parasternal lymph nodes
32 Juxtaesophageal lymph nodes
33 Prevertebral lymph nodes
34 Prepericardial lymph nodes
35 Intercostal lymph nodes
36 Lateral pericardial lymph nodes

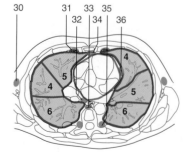

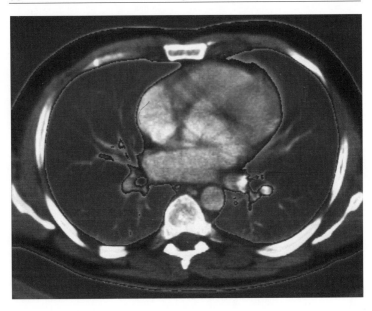

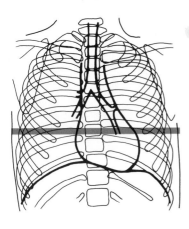

1 Thoracodorsal artery and vein
2 Serratus anterior muscle
3 Pectoralis major muscle
4 Right pulmonary artery
5 Right inferior lobar bronchus
6 Superior vena cava
7 Sternum
8 Right atrium
9 Left atrium
10 Right coronary artery
11 Ascending aorta
12 Internal thoracic artery and vein
13 Left coronary artery
14 Right ventricle
15 Circumflex branch of left coronary artery
16 Left ventricle
17 Right inferior lobar bronchus
18 Subscapularis muscle
19 Latissimus dorsi muscle

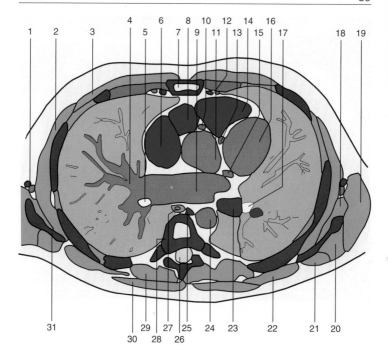

20 Teres major muscle
21 Infraspinatus muscle
22 Rhomboid muscle
23 Left pulmonary artery
24 Descending aorta
25 Azygos vein
26 Spinal canal (dural sac)
27 Esophagus
28 Thoracic vertebra 8
29 Erector spinae muscle
30 Trapezius muscle
31 Scapula
32 Paramammary lymph nodes
33 Lateral pericardial lymph nodes
34 Juxtaesophageal lymph nodes
35 Prepericardial lymph nodes
36 Prevertebral lymph nodes
37 Parasternal lymph nodes
38 Intercostal lymph nodes

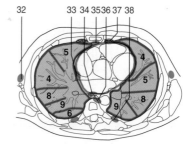

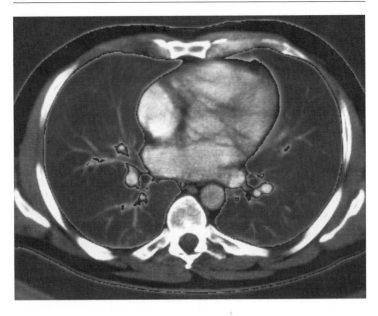

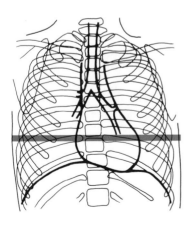

1 Thoracodorsal artery and vein
2 Serratus anterior muscle
3 Pectoralis major muscle
4 Right middle lobar bronchus
5 Right inferior lobar bronchus
6 Internal thoracic artery and vein
7 Superior vena cava
8 Sternum
9 Right atrium
10 Azygos vein
11 Descending aorta
12 Left atrium
13 Right ventricle
14 Right coronary artery
15 Circumflex branch of left coronary
   artery
16 Left ventricle
17 Anterior interventricular branch of
   left coronary artery

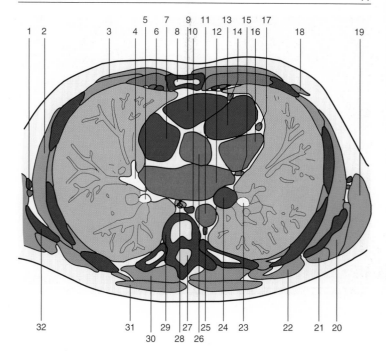

18 Pectoralis minor muscle
19 Latissimus dorsi muscle
20 Teres major muscle
21 Infraspinatus muscle
22 Rhomboid muscle
23 Left inferior lobar bronchus
24 Left pulmonary artery
25 Hemiazygos vein
26 Descending aorta
27 Spinal canal
28 Esophagus
29 Thoracic vertebra 9
30 Erector spinae muscle
31 Trapezius muscle
32 Scapula
33 Paramammary lymph nodes
34 Bronchopulmonary lymph nodes (hilar)
35 Parasternal lymph nodes
36 Prepericardial lymph nodes

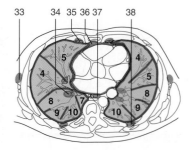

37 Juxtaesophageal lymph nodes
38 Intercostal lymph nodes

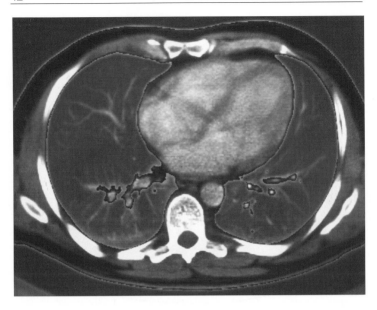

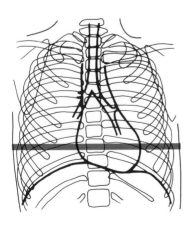

1 Thoracodorsal artery and vein
2 Serratus anterior muscle
3 Right pulmonary vein
4 Right atrium
5 Right coronary artery
6 Sternum
7 Azygos vein
8 Right ventricle
9 Internal thoracic artery and vein
10 Left atrium
11 Left ventricle
12 Anterior interventricular branch of
    left coronary artery
13 Scapula
14 Latissimus dorsi muscle
15 Teres major muscle
16 Infraspinatus muscle
17 Rhomboid muscle
18 Left inferior lobar bronchus

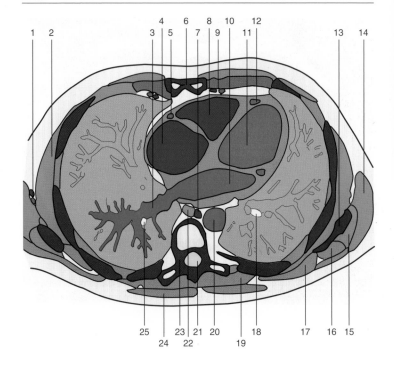

19 Erector spinae muscle
20 Descending aorta
21 Spinal canal
22 Esophagus
23 Thoracic vertebra 9
24 Trapezius muscle
25 Right inferior lobar bronchus
26 Paramammary lymph nodes
27 Intercostal lymph nodes
28 Prevertebral lymph nodes
29 Prepericardial lymph nodes
30 Juxtaesophageal lymph nodes
31 Parasternal lymph nodes
32 Lateral pericardial lymph nodes

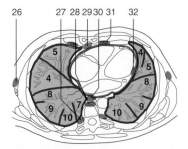

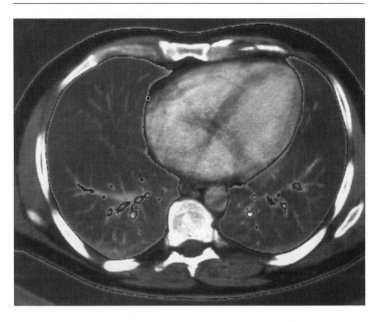

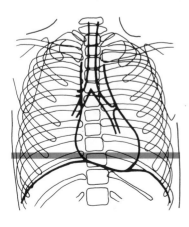

1 Thoracodorsal artery and vein
2 Pectoralis major muscle
3 Right coronary artery
4 Right atrium
5 Sternum
6 Esophagus
7 Azygos vein
8 Right ventricle
9 Descending aorta
10 Internal thoracic artery and vein
11 Circumflex branch of left coronary
   artery
12 Left ventricle
13 Anterior interventricular branch of
   left coronary artery
14 Serratus anterior muscle
15 Latissimus dorsi muscle
16 Scapula
17 Rhomboid muscle

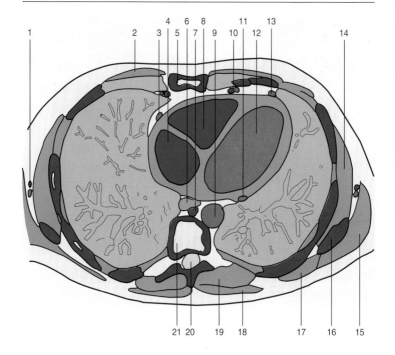

18 Trapezius muscle
19 Erector spinae muscle
20 Spinal canal
21 Thoracic vertebra 9
22 Paramammary lymph nodes
23 Parasternal lymph nodes
24 Prepericardial lymph nodes
25 Prevertebral lymph nodes
26 Juxtaesophageal lymph nodes
27 Intercostal lymph nodes
28 Lateral pericardial lymph nodes

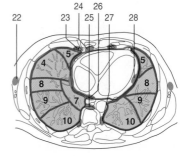

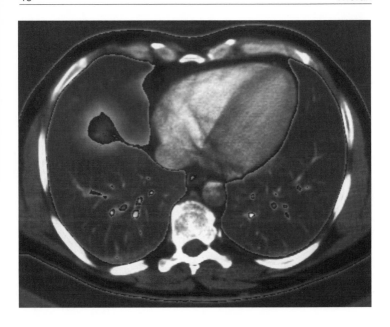

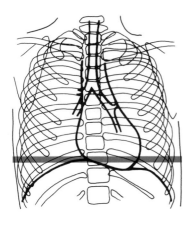

1 Diaphragm
2 Right coronary artery
3 Internal thoracic artery and vein
4 Rectus abdominis muscle
5 Inferior vena cava
6 Sternum
7 Descending aorta
8 Right ventricle
9 Left ventricle
10 Anterior interventricular branch of
   left coronary artery
11 Serratus anterior muscle
12 Latissimus dorsi muscle
13 Coronary sinus
14 Esophagus
15 Azygos vein
16 Spinal canal
17 Thoracic vertebra 10
18 Trapezius muscle

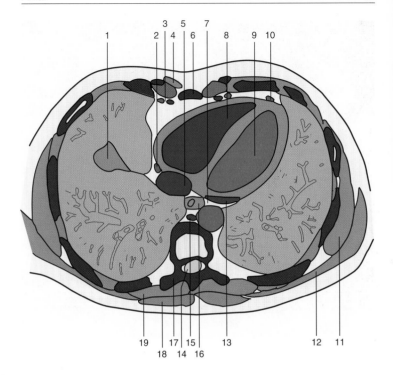

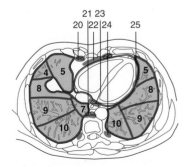

19 Erector spinae muscle
20 Parasternal lymph nodes
21 Prevertebral lymph nodes
22 Prepericardial lymph nodes
23 Superior phrenic lymph nodes
24 Intercostal lymph nodes
25 Lateral pericardial lymph nodes

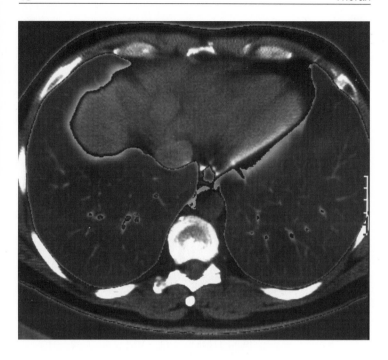

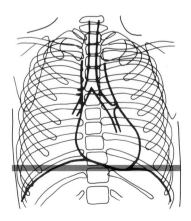

1 External oblique muscle
2 Internal thoracic artery and vein
3 Rectus abdominis muscle
4 Right coronary artery
5 Azygos vein
6 Posterior interventricular branch of
  right coronary artery
7 Sternum
8 Esophagus
9 Hemiazygos vein
10 Right ventricle
11 Left ventricle
12 Anterior interventricular branch of
   left coronary artery
13 Latissimus dorsi muscle
14 Erector spinae muscle
15 Trapezius muscle
16 Descending aorta
17 Spinal canal

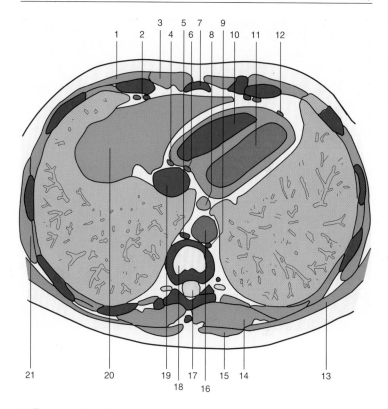

18 Thoracic vertebra 10
19 Inferior vena cava
20 Diaphragm
21 Serratus anterior muscle
22 Parasternal lymph nodes
23 Intercostal lymph nodes
24 Prevertebral lymph nodes
25 Superior phrenic lymph nodes
26 Prepericardial lymph nodes
27 Lateral pericardial lymph nodes

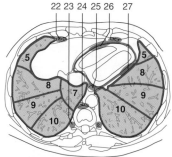

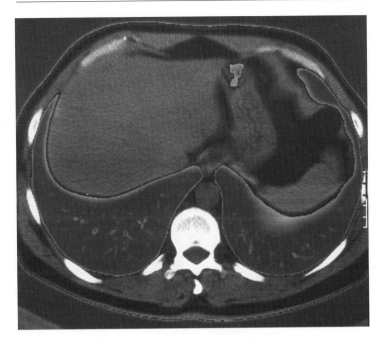

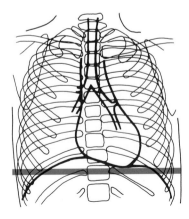

1 External oblique muscle
2 Liver
3 Rectus abdominis muscle
4 Inferior vena cava
5 Internal thoracic artery and vein
6 Azygos vein
7 Esophagus
8 Descending aorta
9 Stomach (fundus)
10 Diaphragm (lumbar part, left crus)
11 Spleen
12 Diaphragm
13 Diaphragm
14 Hemiazygos vein
15 Spinal canal
16 Thoracic vertebra 11
17 Trapezius muscle
18 Erector spinae muscle
19 Latissimus dorsi muscle

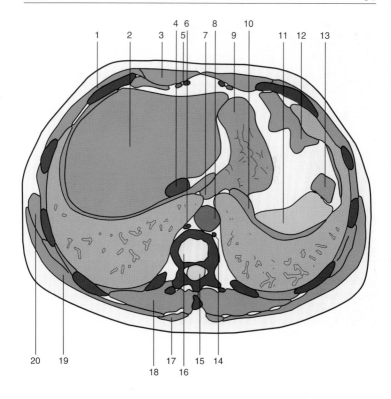

20 Serratus anterior muscle
21 Intercostal lymph nodes
22 Superior phrenic lymph nodes
23 Right gastric lymph nodes
24 Inferior phrenic lymph nodes
25 Left gastroomental lymph nodes

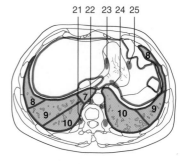

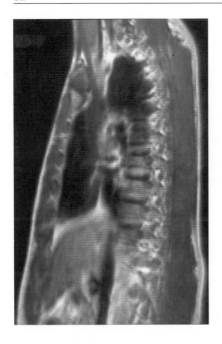

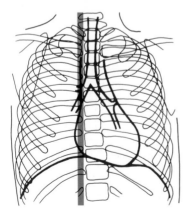

1 Longus colli muscle
2 Thyroid gland
3 Sternocleidomastoid muscle
4 Right common carotid artery
5 External jugular vein
6 Internal jugular vein
7 Clavicle
8 Manubrium of sternum
9 Brachiocephalic vein
10 Pectoralis major muscle
   (clavicular part)
11 Right pulmonary artery
12 Right pulmonary veins
13 Pectoralis major muscle
   (sternocostal part)
14 Right atrium
15 Inferior vena cava
16 Diaphragm
17 Liver
18 Portal vein
19 Rectus abdominis muscle
20 Duodenum
21 Transverse colon
22 Splenius capitis muscle

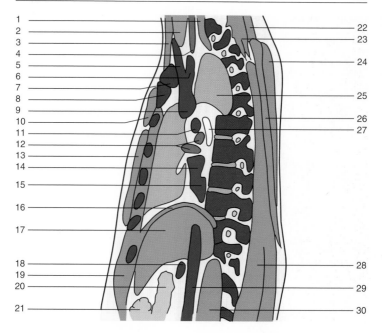

1
2
3
4
5
6
7
8
9
10
11
12
13
14
15
16
17
18
19
20
21

22
23
24
25
26
27
28
29
30

23 Semispinalis capitis muscle
24 Trapezius muscle
25 Right lung
26 Greater rhomboid muscle
27 Right main stem bronchus
28 Erector spinae muscle
29 Inferior vena cava
30 Psoas muscle
31 Thyroid lymph nodes
32 Deep cervical lymph nodes
33 Superficial cervical lymph nodes
34 Bronchopulmonary lymph nodes
35 Prevertebral lymph nodes

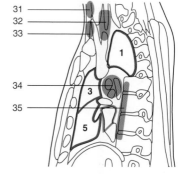

31
32
33

34

35

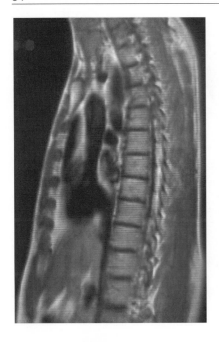

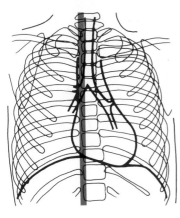

1 Thyroid gland
2 External jugular vein
3 Right common carotid artery
4 Sternocleidomastoid muscle
5 Brachiocephalic trunk
6 Trachea
7 Manubrium of sternum
8 Superior vena cava
9 Pectoralis major muscle (clavicular part)
10 Right lung
11 Right atrial appendage
12 Pectoralis major muscle
     (sternocostal part)
13 Right atrium
14 Liver
15 Pancreas
16 Pylorus
17 Rectus abdominis muscle
18 Transverse colon
19 Splenius capitis muscle
20 Semispinalis capitis muscle
21 Thoracic nerve root
22 Thoracic vertebra 3
23 Trapezius muscle

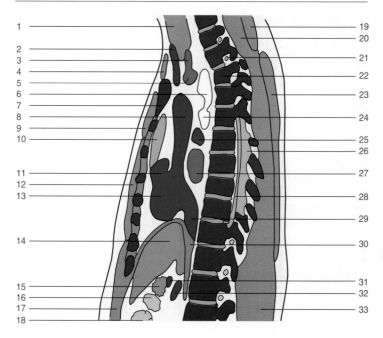

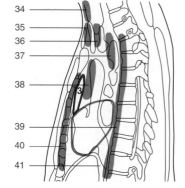

24 Right main stem bronchus
25 Right pulmonary artery
26 Spinal cord
27 Left atrium
28 Dural sac
29 Inferior vena cava
30 Diaphragm
31 Splenic vein
32 Superior mesenteric vein
33 Erector spinae muscle
34 Thyroid lymph nodes
35 Superficial cervical lymph nodes
36 Deep cervical lymph nodes
37 Paratracheal lymph nodes
38 Anterior mediastinal lymph nodes
39 Prevertebral lymph nodes
40 Parasternal lymph nodes
41 Vena caval foramen

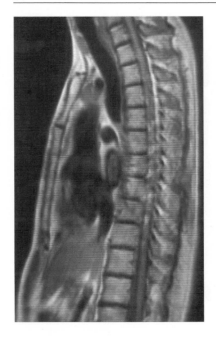

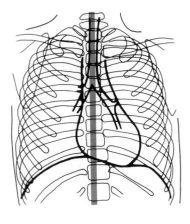

1 Cricoid cartilage
2 Thyroid gland
3 Sternohyoid muscle
4 Jugular venous arch
5 Brachiocephalic trunk
6 Brachiocephalic vein
7 Manubrium of sternum
8 Ascending aorta
9 Sternum (body)
10 Right atrium
11 Right coronary artery
12 Right ventricle
13 Right coronary artery
14 Liver
15 Rectus abdominis muscle
16 Pancreas
17 Pylorus
18 Transverse colon
19 Esophagus
20 Thoracic vertebra 3
21 Trachea
22 Spinal cord
23 Right pulmonary artery
24 Trapezius muscle

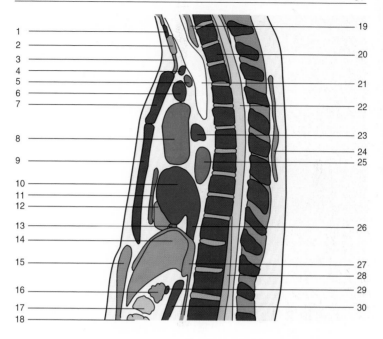

1
2
3
4
5
6
7
8
9
10
11
12
13
14
15
16
17
18

19
20
21
22
23
24
25
26
27
28
29
30

25 Left atrium
26 Inferior vena cava
27 Diaphragm (lumbar part)
28 Dural sac
29 Splenic vein
30 Superior mesenteric vein
31 Pretracheal lymph nodes
32 Paratracheal lymph nodes
33 Anterior mediastinal lymph nodes
34 Inferior tracheobronchial lymph nodes
35 Prevertebral lymph nodes
36 Subpericardial adipose tissue
37 Prepericardial lymph nodes
38 Adipose tissue
39 Superior phrenic lymph nodes

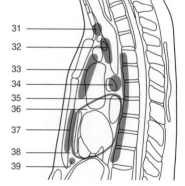

31
32
33
34
35
36
37
38
39

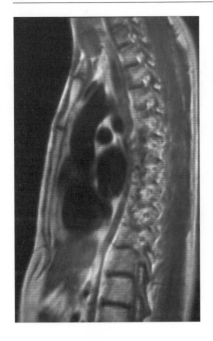

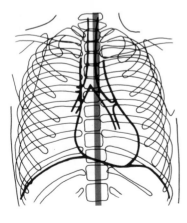

1 Thyroid gland
2 Sternocleidomastoid muscle
3 Jugular venous arch
4 Left brachiocephalic vein
5 Clavicle
6 Internal thoracic vein
7 Aortic arch
8 Manubrium of sternum
9 Ascending aorta
10 Sternum (body)
11 Right coronary artery
12 Right ventricle
13 Diaphragm
14 Liver
15 Rectus abdominis muscle
16 Pancreas
17 Splenic vein
18 Left renal artery
19 Pylorus
20 Inferior mesenteric vein
21 Transverse colon
22 Splenius capitis muscle
23 Semispinalis capitis muscle
24 Nerve root T2

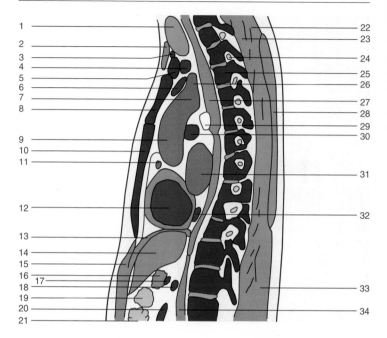

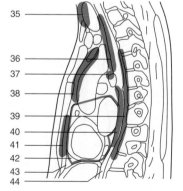

25 Thoracic vertebra 3
26 Brachiocephalic trunk
27 Esophagus
28 Trapezius muscle
29 Left main stem bronchus
30 Right pulmonary artery
31 Left atrium
32 Coronary sinus
33 Erector spinae muscle
34 Diaphragm (lumbar part)
35 Thyroid lymph nodes
36 Paratracheal lymph nodes
37 Superior tracheobronchial lymph nodes
38 Anterior mediastinal lymph nodes
39 Prevertebral lymph nodes
40 Juxtaesophageal lymph nodes
41 Prepericardial lymph nodes
42 Subpericardial adipose tissue
43 Adipose tissue
44 Esophageal hiatus

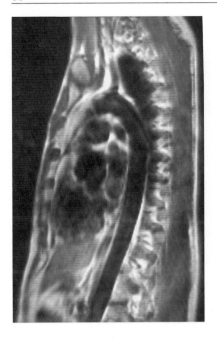

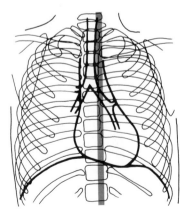

1 Left external carotid artery
2 Left internal carotid artery
3 Sternocleidomastoid muscle
4 Left common carotid artery
5 Internal jugular vein
6 Sternohyoid and sternothyroid muscles
7 Jugular venous arch
8 Clavicle
9 Brachiocephalic vein
10 Manubrium of sternum
11 Pectoralis major muscle
12 Left coronary artery
13 Pulmonary trunk
14 Right ventricle
15 Xyphoid process of sternum
16 Internal thoracic artery
17 Diaphragm
18 Liver
19 Pancreas
20 Rectus abdominis muscle
21 Pylorus
22 Nerve root C8
23 Splenius capitis muscle
24 Semispinalis capitis muscle

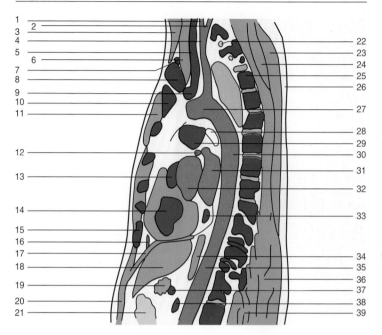

1
2
3
4
5
6
7
8
9
10
11
12
13
14
15
16
17
18
19
20
21

22
23
24
25
26
27
28
29
30
31
32
33
34
35
36
37
38
39

25 Thoracic vertebra 3
26 Trapezius muscle
27 Aortic arch
28 Left main stem bronchus
29 Pulmonary trunk
30 Descending aorta
31 Left atrium
32 Aortic bulb
33 Coronary sinus
34 Diaphragm (lumbar part)
35 Abdominal aorta
36 Erector spinae muscle
37 Splenic vein
38 Left renal vein
39 Quadratus lumborum muscle
40 Deep cervical lymph nodes
41 Aorticopulmonary window
42 Bronchopulmonary lymph nodes
43 Anterior mediastinal lymph nodes
44 Parasternal lymph nodes
45 Subpericardial adipose tissue
46 Pretracheal lymph nodes
47 Adipose tissue

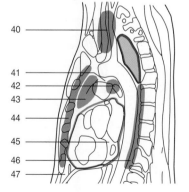

40
41
42
43
44
45
46
47

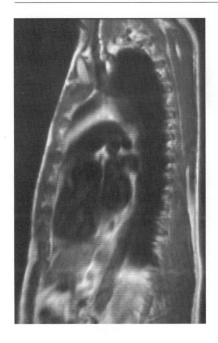

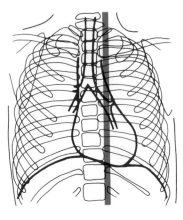

1 Anterior scalene muscle
2 Sternocleidomastoid muscle
3 Internal jugular vein
4 Jugular venous arch
5 Subclavian artery
6 Clavicle
7 Pectoralis major muscle (clavicular part)
8 Left brachiocephalic vein
9 Subclavius muscle
10 Rib 1
11 Pectoralis major muscle
    (sternocostal part)
12 Pulmonary trunk
13 Left pulmonary vein
14 Left coronary artery
15 Aortic bulb
16 Right ventricle
17 Rib 7
18 Liver
19 Stomach
20 Rectus abdominis muscle
21 Pancreas
22 Transverse colon
23 Semispinalis capitis muscle

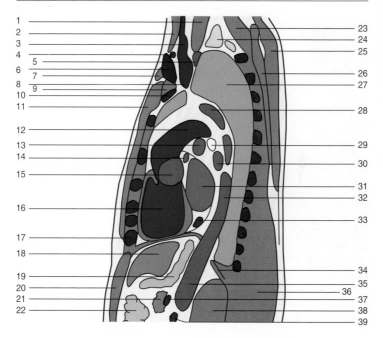

24 Brachial plexus
25 Trapezius muscle
26 Greater rhomboid muscle
27 Left lung
28 Aortic arch
29 Left main stem bronchus
30 Left pulmonary vein
31 Left atrium
32 Descending aorta
33 Coronary sinus
34 Diaphragm
35 Abdominal aorta
36 Erector spinae muscle
37 Splenic vein
38 Psoas muscle
39 Left renal vein
40 Superficial cervical lymph nodes
41 Deep cervical lymph nodes
42 Posterior intercostal lymph nodes
43 Anterior mediastinal lymph nodes
44 Bronchopulmonary lymph nodes
45 Prepericardial lymph nodes
46 Subpericardial adipose tissue
47 Adipose tissue

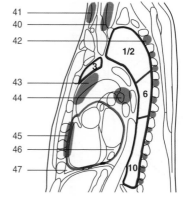

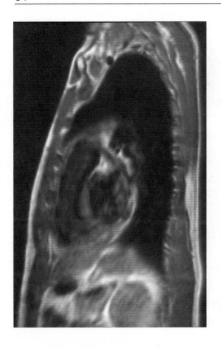

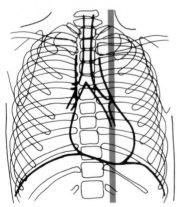

1 Sternocleidomastoid muscle
2 Anterior scalene muscle
3 Left external jugular vein
4 Jugular venous arch
5 Left subclavian artery
6 Sternum
7 Subclavian vein
8 Pectoralis major muscle (sternal part)
9 Subclavius muscle
10 Rib 1
11 Pectoralis major muscle
    (sternocostal part)
12 Left coronary artery
13 Right ventricle
14 Liver (left lobe)
15 Transverse colon
16 Pancreas
17 Rectus abdominis muscle
18 Jejunum
19 Semispinalis capitis muscle
20 Medial scalene muscle
21 Brachial plexus
22 Trapezius muscle
23 Greater rhomboid muscle

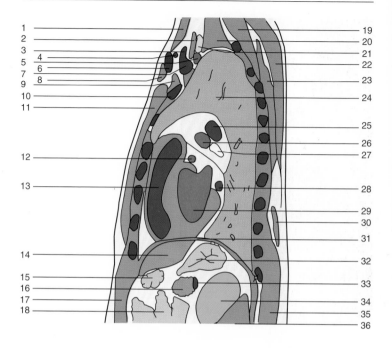

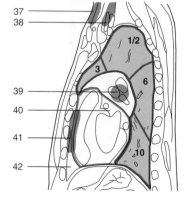

24 Left lung
25 Left pulmonary artery
26 Left pulmonary vein
27 Left main stem bronchus
28 Coronary sinus
29 Left ventricle
30 Latissimus dorsi muscle
31 Diaphragm
32 Stomach
33 Splenic vein
34 Left kidney
35 Erector spinae muscle
36 Psoas muscle
37 Superficial cervical lymph nodes
38 Deep cervical lymph nodes
39 Bronchopulmonary lymph nodes
40 Subpericardial adipose tissue
41 Prepericardial lymph nodes
42 Adipose tissue

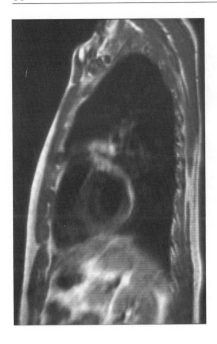

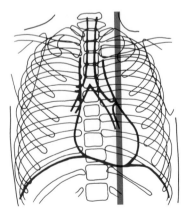

1 Sternocleidomastoid muscle
2 External jugular vein
3 Brachial plexus
4 Clavicle
5 Subclavian artery
6 Subclavian vein
7 Pectoralis major muscle (clavicular part)
8 Subclavius muscle
9 Rib 1
10 Pectoralis major muscle
   (sternocostal part)
11 Left pulmonary artery
12 Right ventricle
13 Liver (left lobe)
14 Rectus abdominis muscle
15 Transverse colon
16 Pancreas
17 Jejunum
18 Levator scapulae muscle
19 Anterior scalene muscle
20 Medial scalene muscle
21 Posterior scalene muscle
22 Scapula
23 Trapezius muscle

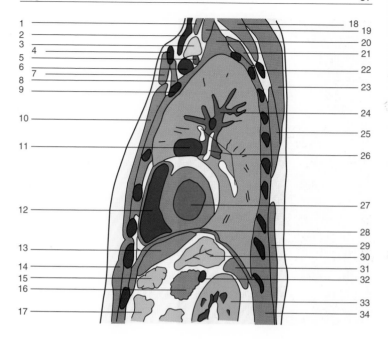

24 Pulmonary arteries
25 Greater rhomboid muscle
26 Segmental bronchi
27 Left ventricle
28 Diaphragm
29 Latissimus dorsi muscle
30 Stomach
31 Spleen
32 Splenic vein
33 Left kidney
34 Erector spinae muscle
35 Superficial cervical lymph nodes
36 Nuchal lymph nodes
37 Supraclavicular lymph nodes
38 Pulmonary lymph nodes
39 Subpericardial adipose tissue
40 Prepericardial lymph nodes

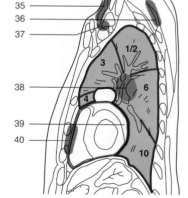

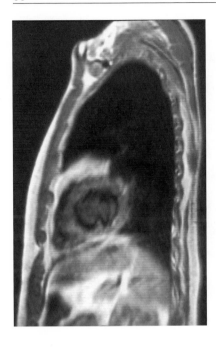

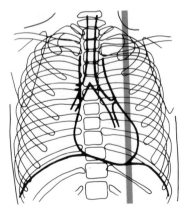

1 Levator scapulae muscle
2 Omohyoid muscle
3 Clavicle
4 Subclavius muscle
5 Subclavian vein
6 Pectoralis major muscle (clavicular part)
7 Rib 1
8 Pectoralis major muscle
    (sternocostal part)
9 Left ventricle
10 Right ventricle
11 Rib 12 (cartilage)
12 Splenic vein
13 Pancreas
14 Jejunum
15 Medial and posterior scalene muscles
16 Scapula
17 Brachial plexus
18 Serratus anterior muscle
19 Subclavian artery
20 Trapezius muscle
21 Greater rhomboid muscle
22 Left lung
23 Diaphragm

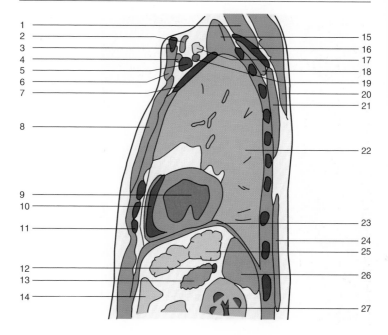

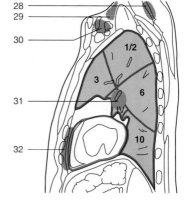

24 Latissimus dorsi muscle
25 Transverse colon
26 Spleen
27 Left kidney
28 Nuchal lymph nodes
29 Superficial cervical lymph nodes
30 Supraclavicular lymph nodes
31 Pulmonary lymph nodes
32 Prepericardial lymph nodes

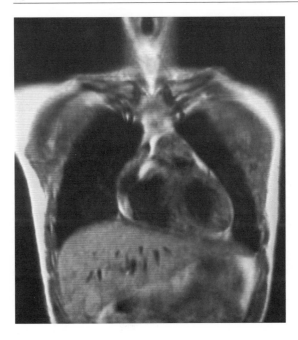

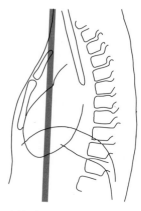

1 Trachea
2 Skin
3 Clavicle
4 Sternocleidomastoid muscle
5 Internal thoracic artery
6 Pectoralis minor muscle

7 Pectoralis major muscle
8 Right coronary artery
9 Right atrial appendage
10 Right lung
11 Right atrium
12 Diaphragm
13 Liver
14 Gall bladder
15 Thyroid cartilage
16 Sternohyoid muscle
17 Pectoralis major muscle (clavicular part)
18 Sternum
19 Internal thoracic vein
20 Pectoralis major muscle
   (sternocostal part)
21 Pulmonary trunk
22 Right lung
23 Left ventricle
24 Transverse colon
25 Descending colon
26 Superficial cervical lymph nodes
27 Anterior mediastinal lymph nodes
28 Lateral pericardial lymph nodes

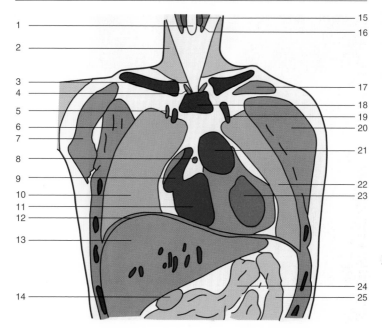

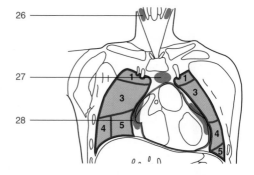

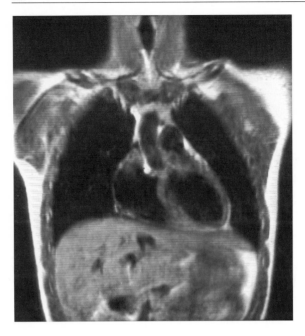

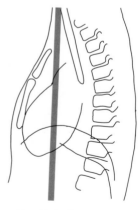

1 Thyroid gland
2 Sternocleidomastoid muscle
   (sternal part)
3 Deltoid muscle
4 Internal thoracic artery and vein
5 Pectoralis minor muscle

6 Pectoralis major muscle
7 Right lung
8 Right atrium
9 Diaphragm
10 Liver (right lobe)
11 Gall bladder
12 Trachea
13 Sternocleidomastoid muscle
   (clavicular part)
14 Clavicle
15 Sternum
16 Skin
17 Descending aorta
18 Pulmonary trunk
19 Left lung
20 Anterior interventricular branch of
   left coronary artery
21 Left ventricle
22 Liver (left lobe)
23 Colon (splenic flexure)
24 Celiac trunk
25 Superior mesenteric artery
26 Transverse colon
27 Superficial cervical lymph nodes

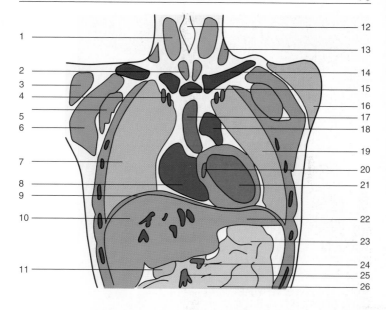

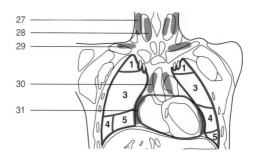

28 Thyroid lymph nodes
29 Supraclavicular lymph nodes
30 Anterior mediastinal lymph nodes
31 Lateral pericardial lymph nodes

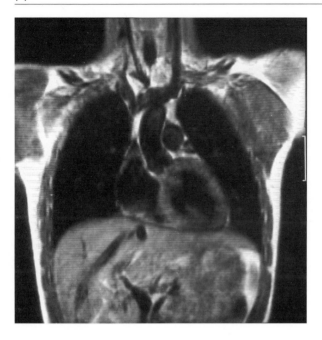

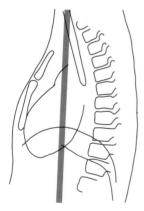

1 Sternocleidomastoid muscle
2 Right common carotid artery
3 Trachea
4 Brachiocephalic trunk
5 Clavicle
6 Right brachiocephalic vein

7 Ascending aorta
8 Superior vena cava
9 Right lung
10 Right atrium
11 Diaphragm
12 Hepatic veins
13 Liver
14 Portal vein
15 Superior mesenteric artery
16 Internal jugular vein
17 Skin
18 Left subclavian vein
19 Internal thoracic artery
20 Left brachiocephalic vein
21 Pectoralis minor muscle
22 Pectoralis major muscle
23 Pulmonary trunk
24 Left atrial appendage
25 Left lung
26 Left atrium
27 Coronary sinus
28 Colon (splenic flexure)
29 Celiac trunk
30 Jejunum

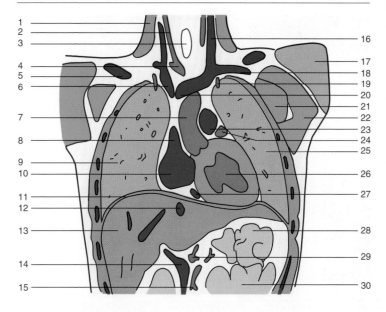

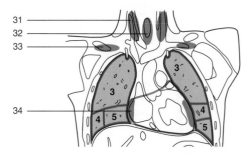

31 Deep cervical lymph nodes
32 Paratracheal lymph nodes
33 Deep axillary lymph nodes
34 Lateral pericardial lymph nodes

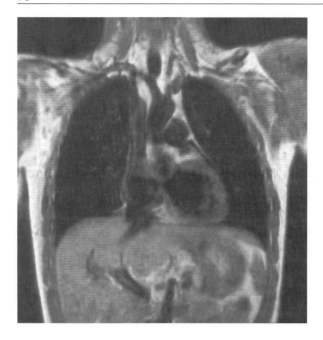

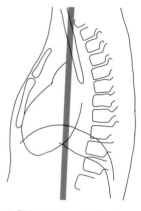

1 Right common carotid artery
2 Esophagus
3 Thyrocervical trunk
4 Subclavian artery
5 Suprascapular artery
6 Deltoid muscle

7 Right brachiocephalic vein
8 Brachiocephalic trunk
9 Serratus anterior muscle
10 Head of humerus
11 Brachial plexus
12 Aortic arch
13 Pectoralis minor muscle
14 Axillary artery and vein
15 Superior vena cava
16 Aortic sinus
17 Right lung
18 Right atrium
19 Diaphragm
20 Hepatic vein
21 Celiac trunk
22 Portal vein
23 Liver (right lobe)
24 Abdominal aorta
25 Sternocleidomastoid muscle
26 Left common carotid artery
27 Anterior scalene muscle
28 Clavicle
29 Trachea
30 Left subclavian artery

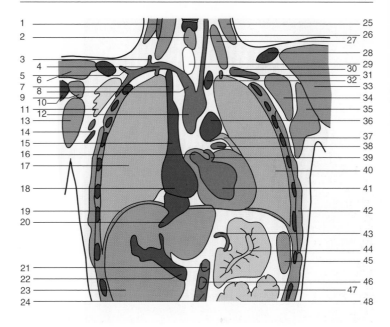

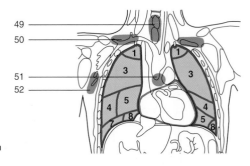

31 Internal thoracic artery
32 Left brachiocephalic vein
33 Deltoid muscle
34 Pectoralis minor muscle
35 Pectoralis major muscle
36 Pulmonary trunk
37 Pericardium
38 Left atrial appendage
39 Left coronary artery
40 Left lung
41 Left ventricle
42 Serratus anterior muscle
43 Left gastric artery

44 Stomach
45 Spleen
46 Superior mesenteric artery
47 Colon (splenic flexure)
48 Transverse colon
49 Paratracheal lymph nodes
50 Deep axillary lymph nodes
51 Anterior mediastinal lymph nodes
52 Superficial axillary lymph nodes

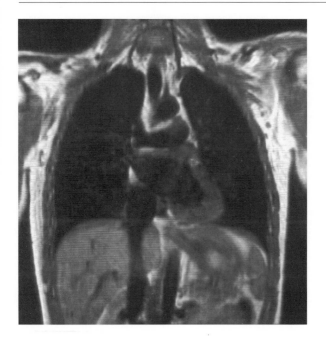

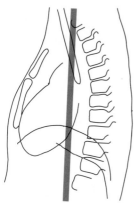

1 Spinal cord
2 Dural sac
3 Sternocleidomastoid muscle
4 Thoracic vertebra 1
5 Medial scalene muscle
6 Superficial cervical artery

7 Clavicle
8 Brachial plexus
9 Head of humerus
10 Axillary artery
11 Axillary vein
12 Pulmonary trunk
13 Right atrium
14 Serratus anterior muscle
15 Diaphragm
16 Inferior vena cava
17 Liver
18 Abdominal aorta
19 Left renal vein
20 Duodenum
21 Portal vein
22 Left vertebral artery
23 Brachial plexus
24 Deltoid muscle
25 Omohyoid muscle
26 Coracoid process
27 Left subclavian artery
28 Pectoralis minor muscle
29 Trachea
30 Left common carotid artery

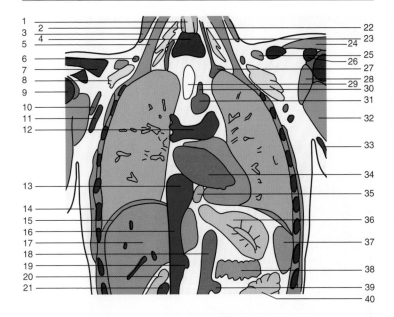

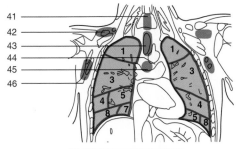

31 Aortic arch
32 Triceps muscle
33 Axillary vein
34 Left ventricle
35 Esophagus
36 Stomach
37 Spleen
38 Pancreas

39 Inferior mesenteric artery
40 Splenic flexure of colon
41 Prevertebral lymph nodes
42 Deep axillary lymph nodes
43 Paratracheal lymph nodes
44 Aorticopulmonary window
45 Tracheobronchial lymph nodes
46 Superficial axillary lymph nodes

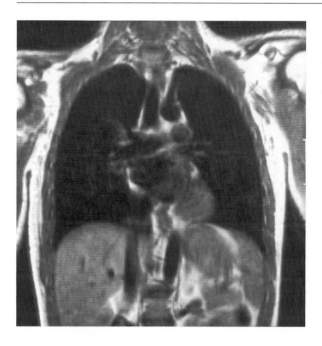

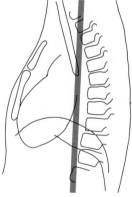

1 Spinal cord
2 Spinal canal
3 Brachial plexus
4 Superficial cervical artery
5 Trapezius muscle
6 Axillary nerve
7 Serratus anterior muscle

8 Head of humerus
9 Subscapularis muscle
10 Aortic arch
11 Trachea
12 Pulmonary trunk
13 Right pulmonary artery
14 Left atrium
15 Triceps muscle
16 Esophagus
17 Liver (right lobe)
18 Latissimus dorsi muscle
19 Diaphragm (lumbar part)
20 Inferior vena cava
21 Liver (caudate lobe)
22 Duodenum
23 Right kidney
24 Medial scalene muscle
25 Sternocleidomastoid muscle
26 Clavicle
27 Suprascapular vein
28 Coracoid process
29 Thoracic vertebra 2
30 Left subclavian artery
31 Esophagus
32 Median nerve

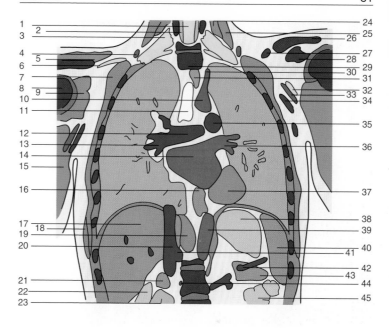

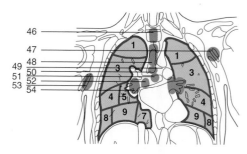

33 Axillary artery
34 Axillary vein
35 Left pulmonary artery
36 Left pulmonary vein
37 Left ventricle (muscle)
38 Stomach (fundus)
39 Abdominal aorta
40 Spleen
41 Left renal vein
42 Splenic vein
43 Pancreas

44 Intercostal artery
45 Transverse colon
46 Prevertebral lymph nodes
47 Deep axillary lymph nodes
48 Paratracheal lymph nodes
49 Aorticopulmonary window
50 Superior tracheobronchial lymph nodes
51 Inferior tracheobronchial lymph nodes
52 Bronchopulmonary lymph nodes
53 Superficial axillary lymph nodes
54 Pulmonary lymph nodes

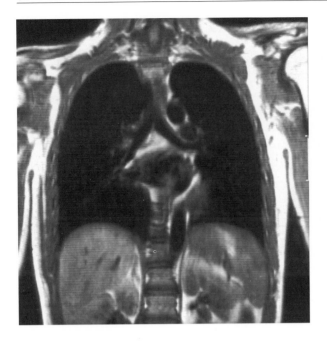

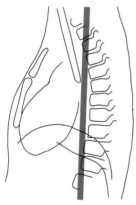

1 Spinal cord
2 Vertebral artery
3 Nerve root pocket
4 Brachial plexus
5 Superficial cervical artery
6 Thoracic vertebra 2

7 Head of humerus
8 Trachea
9 Aortic arch
10 Left pulmonary artery
11 Right superior lobar bronchus
12 Right pulmonary artery
13 Right inferior lobar bronchus
14 Left atrium
15 Latissimus dorsi muscle
16 Diaphragm
17 Liver
18 Right adrenal gland
19 Liver (caudate lobe)
20 Right kidney
21 Sternocleidomastoid muscle
22 Medial scalene muscle
23 Clavicle
24 Supraspinatus tendon
25 Coracoid process
26 Serratus anterior muscle
27 Subscapularis muscle
28 Esophagus
29 Median nerve
30 Axillary artery

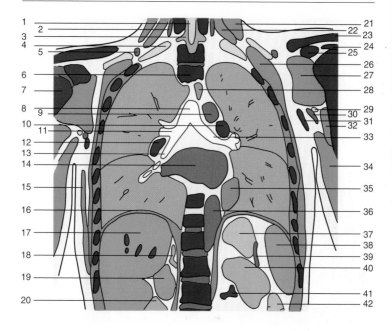

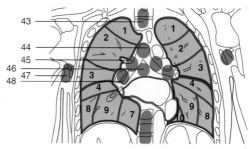

31 Axillary vein
32 Coracobrachialis muscle
33 Left main stem bronchus
34 Biceps muscle
35 Left ventricle (muscle)
36 Abdominal aorta
37 Stomach (fundus)
38 Spleen
39 Gastroepiploic artery
40 Left kidney

41 Left renal vein
42 Descending colon
43 Prevertebral lymph nodes
44 Superior tracheobronchial lymph
   nodes
45 Bronchopulmonary lymph nodes
46 Inferior tracheobronchial lymph nodes
47 Superficial axillary lymph nodes
48 Pulmonary lymph nodes

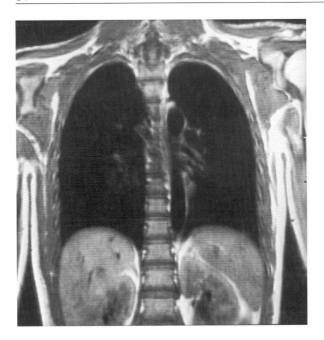

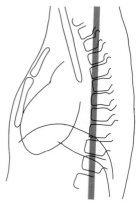

1 Trapezius muscle
2 Superficial cervical artery
3 Brachial plexus
4 Supraspinatus muscle
5 Serratus anterior muscle
6 Neck of scapula

7 Head of humerus
8 Subscapularis muscle
9 Right lung
10 Teres major muscle
11 Intercostal artery
12 Latissimus dorsi muscle
13 Brachial artery
14 Liver (right lobe)
15 Erector spinae muscle
16 Clavicle
17 Spinal cord
18 Cervical interspinal muscles
19 Dural sac
20 Thoracic vertebra 2
21 Glenoid lip
22 Teres major muscle
23 Left lung
24 Aortic arch
25 Esophagus
26 Left pulmonary artery
27 Pulmonary veins
28 Descending aorta
29 Latissimus dorsi muscle
30 Biceps muscle

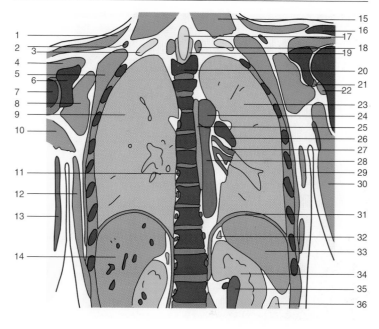

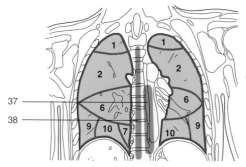

31 Diaphragm
32 Left adrenal gland
33 Spleen
34 Left kidney
35 Renal pelvis
36 Descending colon
37 Juxtaesophageal lymph nodes
38 Prevertebral lymph nodes

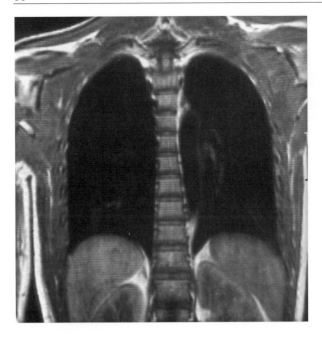

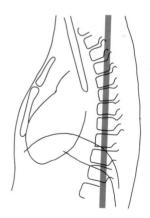

1 Spinous process of cervical vertebra 7
2 Trapezius muscle
3 Levator scapulae muscle
4 Root of spinal nerve T2
5 Spine of scapula
6 Thoracic vertebra 3

7 Lateral margin of scapula
8 Right lung
9 Latissimus dorsi muscle
10 Intervertebral artery
11 Triceps muscle
12 Brachial artery
13 Liver
14 Right adrenal gland
15 Right kidney
16 Erector spinae muscle
17 Superficial cervical artery
18 Supraspinatus muscle
19 Dural sac
20 Spinal cord
21 Infraspinatus muscle
22 Subscapularis muscle
23 Serratus anterior muscle
24 Teres major muscle
25 Descending aorta
26 Left pulmonary artery
27 Left lung
28 Diaphragm
29 Spleen

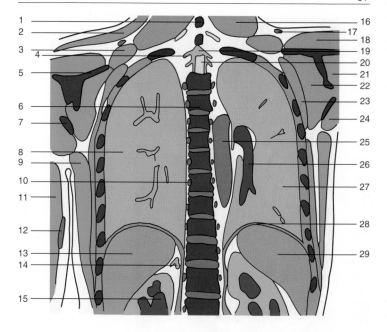

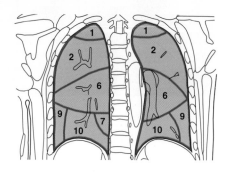

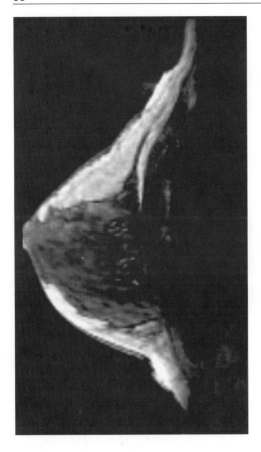

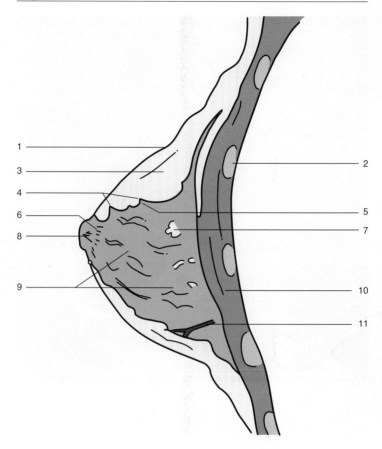

1 Skin
2 Rib
3 Subcutaneous adipose tissue
4 Margins of glandular lobes
5 Suspensory ligaments of Cooper
6 Retromamillary space with lactiferous
   ducts

7 Adipose tissue
8 Nipple
9 Glandular tissue
10 Pectoralis muscle
11 Vein

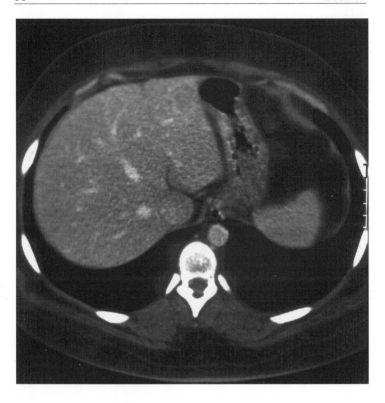

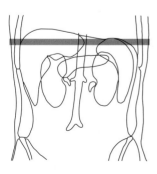

1 Liver
2 Rectus abdominis muscle
3 Inferior vena cava
4 Liver (left lobe)
5 Azygos vein
6 Esophagus
7 Stomach
8 Diaphragm
9 Left lung
10 Spleen
11 Diaphragm (lumbar part)
12 Abdominal aorta
13 Hemiazygos vein
14 Spinalis muscle

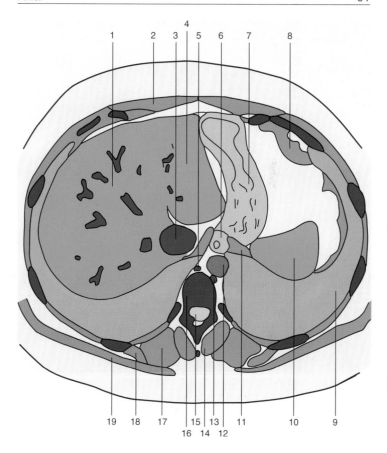

15 Spinal canal
16 Thoracic vertebra 9
17 Longissimus thoracis muscle
18 Iliocostalis lumborum muscle
19 Latissimus dorsi muscle
20 Intercostal lymph nodes
21 Superior phrenic lymph nodes
22 Inferior phrenic lymph nodes
23 Gastroomental lymph nodes

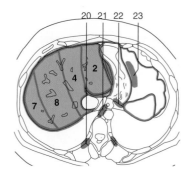

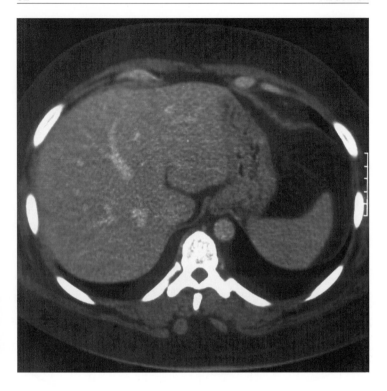

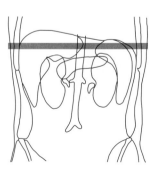

1 Right hepatic vein
2 Rectus abdominis muscle
3 Inferior vena cava
4 Liver (left lobe)
5 Azygos vein
6 Abdominal aorta
7 Stomach
8 Diaphragm
9 Serratus anterior muscle
10 Latissimus dorsi muscle
11 Spleen
12 Hemiazygos vein
13 Spinalis muscle
14 Thoracic vertebra 9

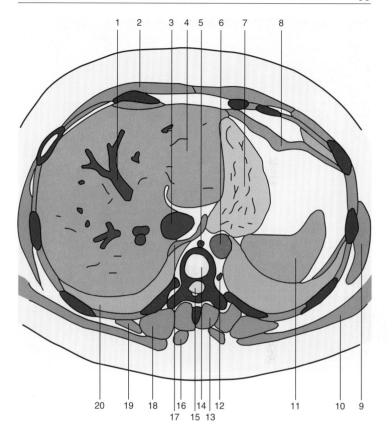

15 Spinal canal
16 Trapezius muscle
17 Diaphragm
18 Longissimus thoracis muscle
19 Iliocostalis lumborum muscle
20 Right lung
21 Intercostal lymph nodes
22 Superior phrenic lymph nodes
23 Right gastric lymph nodes
24 Inferior phrenic lymph nodes
25 Gastroomental lymph nodes

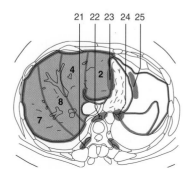

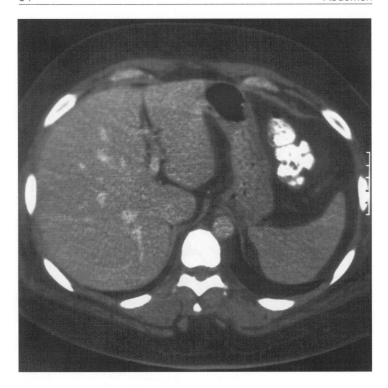

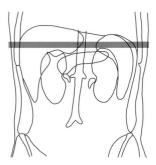

1 External oblique muscle
2 Liver (right lobe)
3 Rectus abdominis muscle
4 Portal vein
5 Liver (left lobe)
6 Inferior vena cava
7 Diaphragm

8 Azygos vein
9 Right inferior phrenic artery
10 Left inferior phrenic artery
11 Common hepatic artery
12 Splenic artery
13 Stomach
14 Short gastric artery
15 Transverse colon
16 Spleen
17 Left lung
18 Left inferior phrenic artery
19 Hemiazygos vein
20 Abdominal aorta
21 Spinal canal
22 Thoracic vertebra 10
23 Spinalis muscle
24 Liver (caudate lobe)
25 Longissimus thoracis muscle
26 Iliocostalis thoracis muscle
27 Latissimus dorsi muscle
28 Intercostal lymph nodes

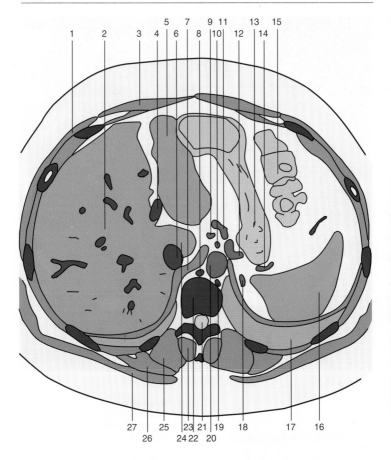

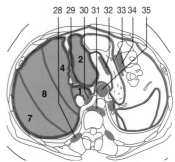

29 Hepatic lymph nodes
30 Inferior phrenic lymph nodes
31 Superior phrenic lymph nodes
32 Right gastric lymph nodes
33 Gastroomental lymph nodes
34 Paracolic lymph nodes
35 Celiac lymph nodes

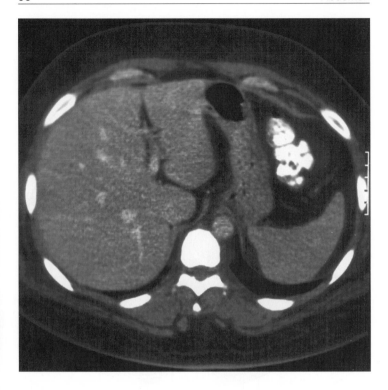

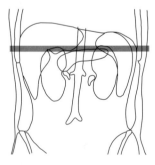

1 Liver
2 Rectus abdominis muscle
3 Portal vein
4 Liver (left lobe)
5 Liver (caudate lobe)
6 Inferior vena cava
7 Linea alba

8 Azygos vein
9 Abdominal aorta
10 Hemiazygos vein
11 Diaphragm
12 Stomach
13 Diaphragm
14 External oblique muscle
15 Splenic flexure of colon
16 Serratus anterior muscle
17 Latissimus dorsi muscle
18 Spleen
19 Left lung
20 Spinal nerve root T10
21 Spinalis muscle
22 Spinal canal
23 Thoracic vertebra 10
24 Longissimus thoracis muscle
25 Iliocostalis thoracis muscle
26 Diaphragm
27 Hepatic lymph nodes
28 Inferior phrenic lymph nodes

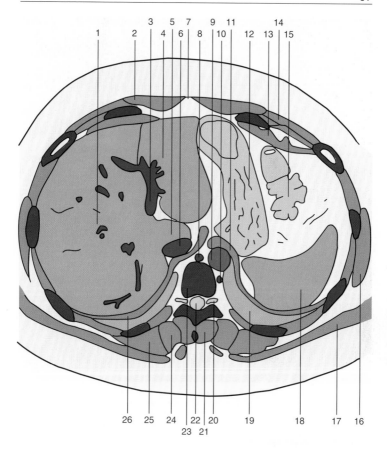

29 Inferior phrenic lymph nodes
30 Right gastric lymph nodes
31 Gastroomental lymph nodes
32 Intercostal lymph nodes

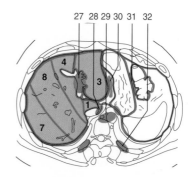

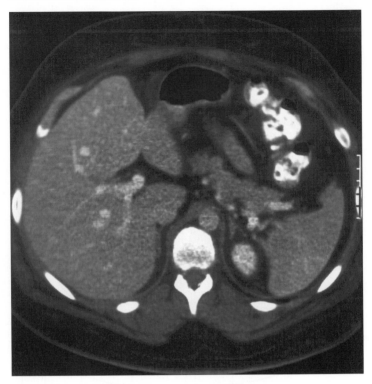

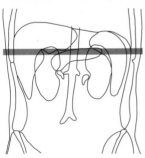

1 External oblique muscle
2 Liver (right lobe)
3 Rectus abdominis muscle
4 Left gastric artery and vein
5 Liver (left lobe)
6 Inferior vena cava
7 Stomach

8 Right gastric artery
9 Azygos vein
10 Abdominal aorta
11 Jejunum
12 Middle colic vein
13 Pancreas
14 Splenic vein
15 Transverse colon
16 Splenic flexure of colon
17 Spleen
18 Latissimus dorsi muscle
19 Left lung, costodiaphragmatic recess
20 Left kidney
21 Left adrenal gland
22 Longissimus thoracis muscle
23 Hemiazygos vein
24 Thoracic vertebra 11
25 Spinal canal
26 Diaphragm
27 Spinalis muscle
28 Spinal nerve root T 10

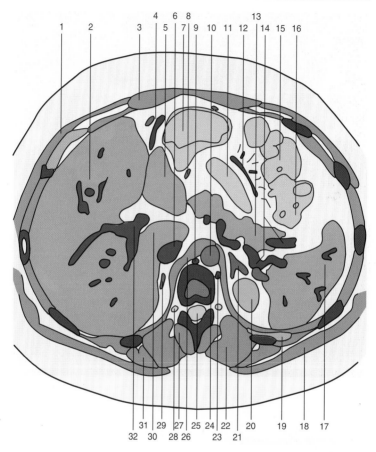

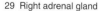

29 Right adrenal gland
30 Liver (caudate lobe)
31 Iliocostalis thoracis muscle
32 Portal vein
33 Intercostal lymph node
34 Hepatic lymph nodes
35 Right gastric lymph nodes
36 Superior phrenic lymph nodes
37 Gastroomental lymph nodes
38 Paracolic lymph nodes
39 Pancreatic lymph nodes
40 Pancreatic lymph nodes
41 Splenic lymph nodes

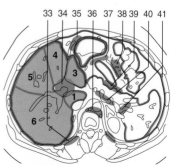

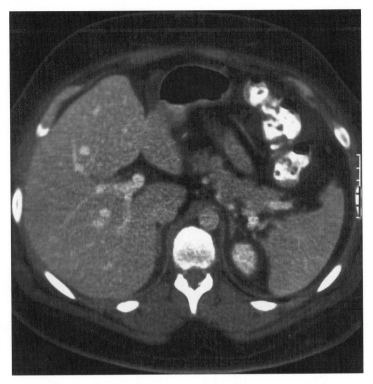

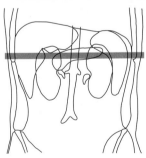

8 Abdominal aorta
9 Jejunum
10 Splenic vein
11 Transverse colon
12 Splenic artery
13 Splenic flexure of colon
14 Spleen
15 Left lung
16 Inferior posterior serratus anterior
    muscle
17 Iliocostalis thoracis muscle
18 Left adrenal gland
19 Spinalis muscle
20 Spinal canal
21 Thoracic vertebra 11
22 Diaphragm
23 Longissimus thoracis muscle
24 Right kidney
25 Latissimus dorsi muscle
26 Liver
27 Intercostal lymph nodes
28 Hepatic lymph nodes

1 External oblique muscle
2 Rectus abdominis muscle
3 Portal vein
4 Stomach
5 Inferior vena cava
6 Left gastric artery
7 Pancreas

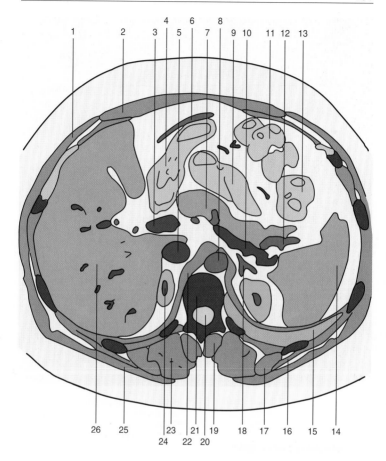

29 Right gastric lymph nodes
30 Lumbar lymph nodes
31 Gastroomental lymph nodes
32 Pancreatic lymph nodes
33 Paracolic lymph nodes
34 Superior phrenic lymph nodes
35 Splenic lymph nodes

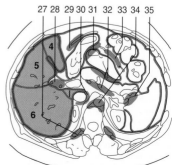

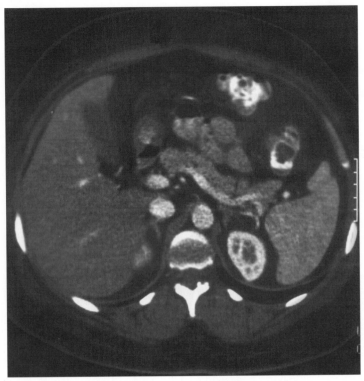

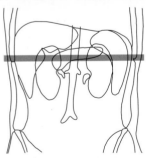

8 Left gastric artery and vein
9 Jejunum
10 Abdominal aorta
11 Splenic vein
12 Pancreas
13 Transverse colon
14 Splenic artery
15 Descending colon
16 Internal oblique muscle
17 Spleen
18 Left lung (costodiaphragmatic recess)
19 Inferior posterior serratus anterior
   muscle
20 Left renal cortex
21 Iliocostalis thoracis muscle
22 Renal medulla
23 Left adrenal gland
24 Longissimus thoracis muscle
25 Spinalis muscle
26 Spinal canal
27 Thoracic vertebra 11

1 External oblique muscle
2 Liver
3 Gall bladder
4 Rectus abdominis muscle
5 Ampulla of duodenum
6 Duodenum
7 Inferior vena cava

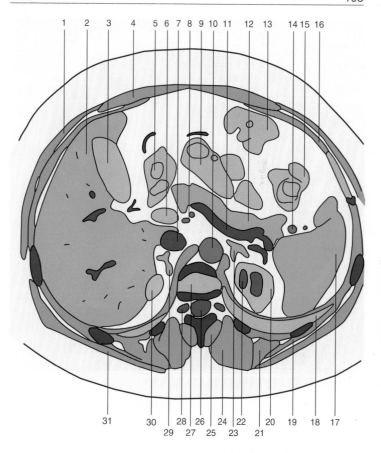

28 Spinal nerve root T 11
29 Right adrenal gland
30 Right kidney
31 Latissimus dorsi muscle
32 Cystic lymph nodes
33 Hepatic lymph nodes
34 Intercostal lymph nodes
35 Gastroomental lymph nodes
36 Lumbar lymph nodes
37 Superior phrenic lymph nodes
38 Pancreatic lymph nodes
39 Left lumbar lymph nodes
40 Juxtaintestinal lymph nodes
41 Paracolic lymph nodes

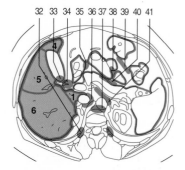

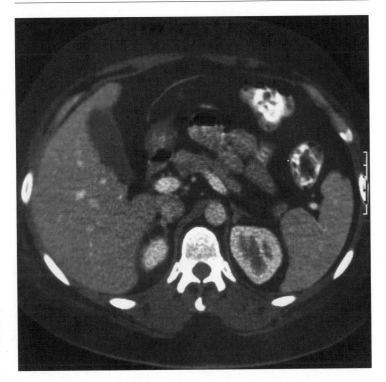

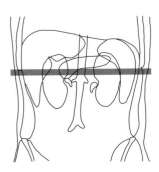

8 Left gastric artery
9 Left gastric artery and vein
10 Stomach
11 Pancreas (body)
12 Splenic vein
13 Right gastric artery
14 Abdominal aorta
15 Jejunum
16 Transverse colon
17 Descending colon
18 Splenic artery
19 Spleen
20 Latissimus dorsi muscle
21 Inferior posterior serratus anterior muscle
22 Left renal cortex
23 Iliocostalis thoracis muscle
24 Renal medulla
25 Left adrenal gland
26 Thoracic vertebra 12
27 Spinal canal
28 Spinalis muscle

1 External oblique muscle
2 Liver
3 Gall bladder
4 Rectus abdominis muscle
5 Ampulla of duodenum
6 Duodenum (descending part)
7 Inferior vena cava

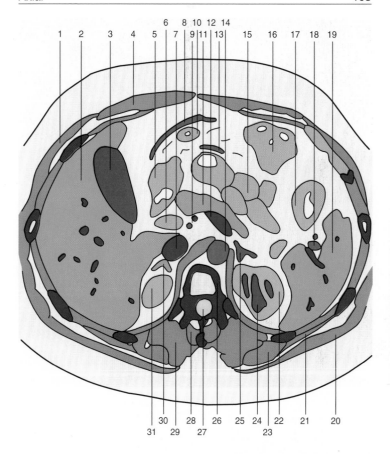

29 Longissimus thoracis muscle
30 Adrenal gland
31 Right kidney
32 Intercostal lymph nodes
33 Lumbar lymph nodes
34 Gastroomental lymph nodes
35 Superior phrenic lymph nodes
36 Pancreatic lymph nodes
37 Paracolic lymph nodes
38 Left lumbar lymph nodes
39 Paracolic lymph nodes

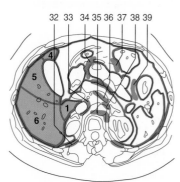

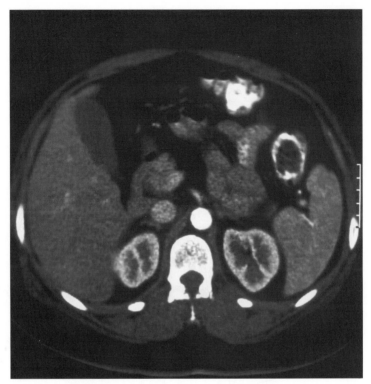

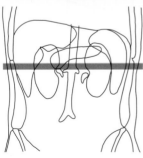

1 External oblique muscle
2 Liver
3 Gall bladder
4 Rectus abdominis muscle
5 Duodenum
6 Pancreas (head)
7 Inferior vena cava

8 Splenic vein
9 Diaphragm
10 Superior mesenteric artery
11 Abdominal aorta
12 Left adrenal gland
13 Jejunum
14 Transverse colon
15 Descending colon
16 Splenic artery
17 Internal oblique muscle
18 Spleen
19 Inferior posterior serratus anterior muscle
20 Renal medulla
21 Iliocostalis thoracis muscle
22 Left renal cortex
23 Longissimus thoracis muscle
24 Thoracic vertebra 12
25 Spinal canal
26 Spinalis muscle
27 Spinal nerve root T11
28 Right adrenal gland

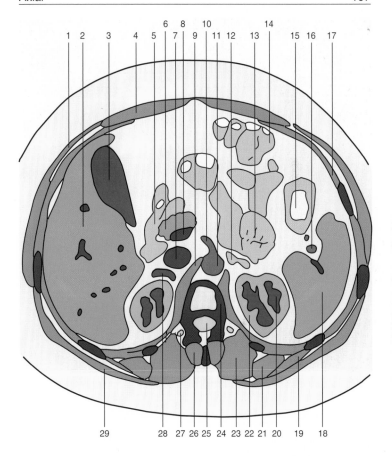

29 Latissimus dorsi muscle
30 Lumbar lymph nodes
31 Pancreatic lymph nodes
32 Juxtaintestinal lymph nodes
33 Superior phrenic lymph nodes
34 Paracolic lymph nodes
35 Superior mesenteric lymph nodes
36 Left lumbar lymph nodes
37 Paracolic lymph nodes
38 Intercostal lymph nodes

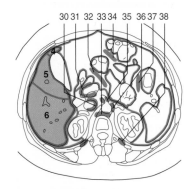

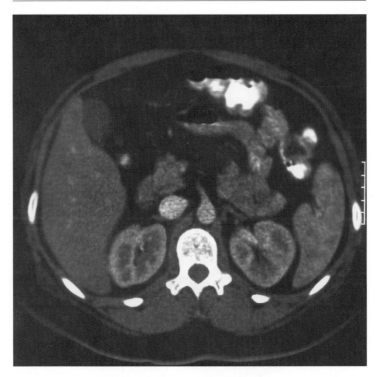

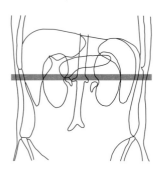

1 External oblique muscle
2 Liver
3 Gall bladder
4 Duodenum (descending part)
5 Middle colic vein
6 Pancreas (head)
7 Inferior vena cava

8 Jejunum
9 Superior mesenteric artery
10 Abdominal aorta
11 Rectus abdominis muscle
12 Renal vein
13 Jejunum
14 Transverse colon
15 Descending colon
16 Splenic artery
17 Internal oblique muscle
18 Latissimus dorsi muscle
19 Spleen
20 Inferior posterior serratus anterior muscle
21 Iliocostalis lumborum muscle
22 Longissimus thoracis muscle
23 Diaphragm
24 Thoracic vertebra 12
25 Spinal canal
26 Spinalis muscle
27 Renal medulla
28 Renal calix

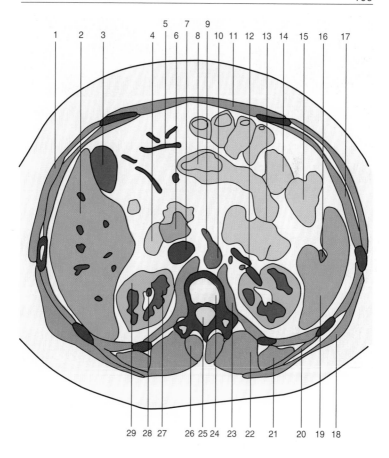

29 Right kidney (renal cortex)
30 Pancreatic lymph nodes
31 Lumbar lymph nodes
32 Superior mesenteric lymph nodes
33 Juxtaintestinal lymph nodes
34 Paracolic lymph nodes
35 Left lumbar lymph nodes

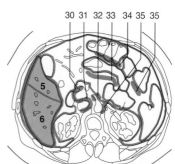

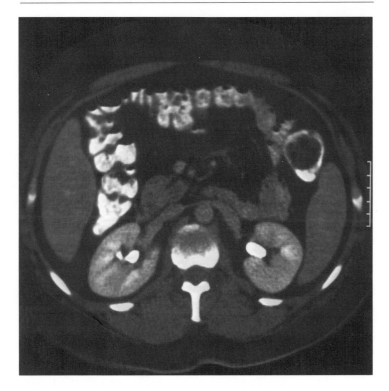

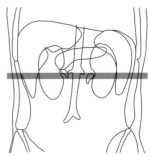

1 Internal oblique muscle
2 External oblique muscle
3 Liver
4 Ascending colon
5 Rectus abdominis muscle
6 Transverse colon
7 Duodenum (descending part)

8 Superior mesenteric vein
9 Superior mesenteric artery
10 Abdominal aorta
11 Left renal vein
12 Middle colic vein
13 Duodenum (inferior horizontal part)
14 Jejunum
15 Descending colon
16 Transversus abdominis muscle
17 Spleen
18 Renal pyramids
19 Left kidney
20 Renal pelvis
21 Longissimus thoracis muscle
22 Diaphragm
23 Lumbar vertebra 1
24 Spinal canal
25 Spinalis muscle
26 Spinal nerve root T12
27 Inferior vena cava
28 Iliocostalis lumborum muscle

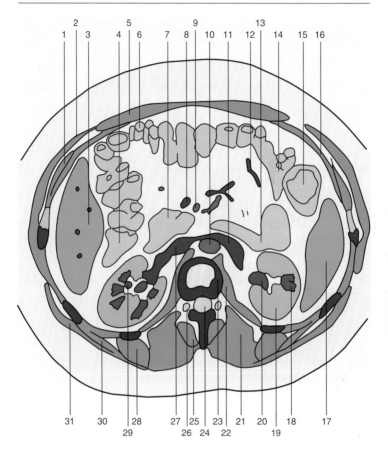

29 Renal calix
30 Inferior posterior serratus anterior muscle
31 Latissimus dorsi muscle
32 Paracolic lymph nodes
33 Pancreatic-duodenal lymph nodes
34 Lumbar lymph nodes
35 Left lumbar lymph nodes
36 Juxtaintestinal lymph nodes

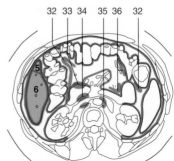

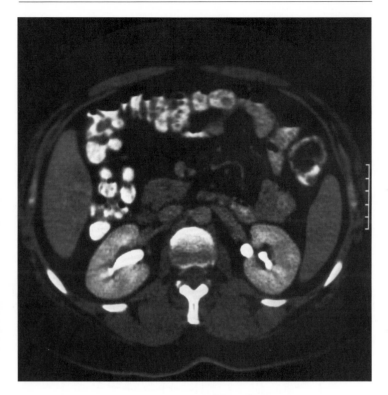

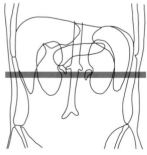

1 Internal oblique muscle
2 Liver
3 Transversus abdominis muscle
4 Transverse colon
5 Right renal artery
6 Duodenum (descending part)
7 Inferior vena cava

8 Superior mesenteric vein
9 Superior mesenteric artery
10 Abdominal aorta
11 Middle colic artery
12 Duodenum (inferior horizontal part)
13 Descending colon
14 Spleen
15 External oblique muscle
16 Inferior posterior serratus anterior muscle
17 Left kidney
18 Renal calix
19 Ureter
20 Left renal vein
21 Longissimus thoracis muscle
22 Spinal nerve root
23 Lumbar vertebra 1
24 Spinal canal
25 Spinalis muscle
26 Diaphragm
27 Psoas muscle
28 Quadratus lumborum muscle

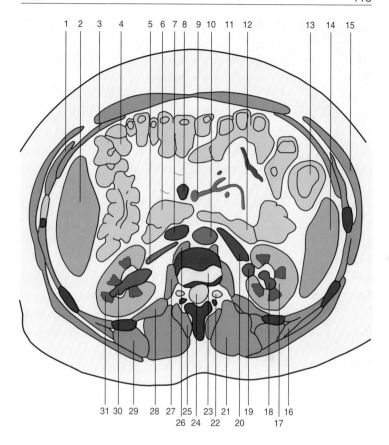

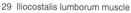

29 Iliocostalis lumborum muscle
30 Renal pelvis
31 Renal pyramid
32 Lumbar lymph nodes
33 Paracolic lymph nodes
34 Inferior pancreatic-duodenal lymph nodes
35 Intermediate lumbar lymph nodes
36 Left lumbar lymph nodes
37 Juxtaintestinal lymph nodes

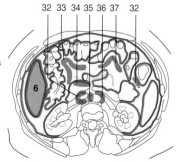

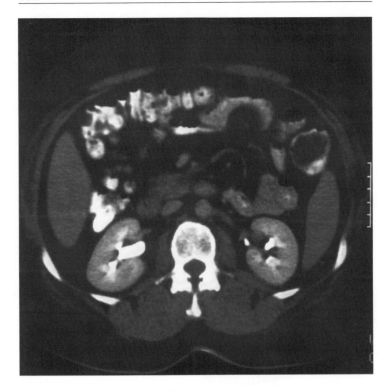

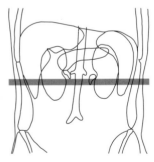

8 Diaphragm
9 Superior mesenteric artery
10 Abdominal aorta
11 Jejunal arteries
12 Left renal artery
13 Ileum
14 Jejunum
15 Descending colon
16 Spleen
17 Internal oblique muscle
18 Transversus abdominis muscle
19 Latissimus dorsi muscle
20 Left kidney
21 Renal calix
22 Renal vein
23 Quadratus lumborum muscle
24 Spinalis muscle
25 Spinal canal
26 Lumbar vertebra 2
27 Psoas muscle
28 Longissimus thoracis muscle

1 Internal oblique muscle
2 Liver
3 Transverse colon
4 Rectus abdominis muscle
5 Duodenum
6 Inferior vena cava
7 Superior mesenteric vein

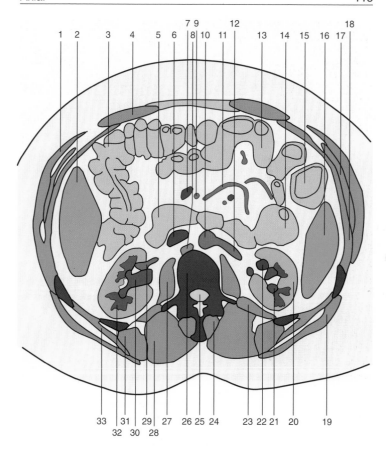

29 Right renal artery
30 Renal pelvis
31 Iliocostalis lumborum muscle
32 Renal pyramid
33 Inferior posterior serratus anterior muscle
34 Paracolic lymph nodes
35 Lumbar lymph nodes
36 Pancreatic-duodenal lymph nodes
37 Intermediate lumbar lymph nodes
38 Superior mesenteric lymph nodes
39 Juxtaintestinal lymph nodes

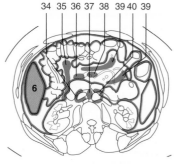

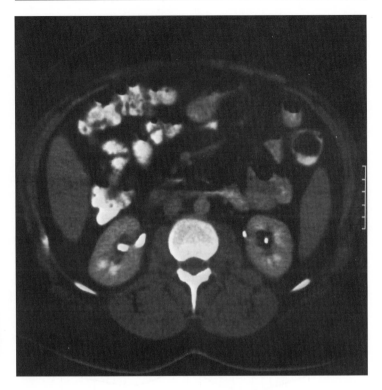

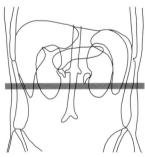

1 External oblique muscle
2 Liver
3 Transversus abdominis muscle
4 Transverse colon
5 Rectus abdominis muscle
6 Duodenum
7 Inferior vena cava

8 Abdominal aorta
9 Jejunal arteries and veins
10 Ileum
11 Descending colon
12 Spleen
13 Internal oblique muscle
14 Latissimus dorsi muscle
15 Left kidney
16 Quadratus lumborum muscle
17 Ureter
18 Psoas muscle
19 Spinalis muscle
20 Spinal canal
21 Lumbar vertebra 2
22 Longissimus thoracis muscle
23 Iliocostalis lumborum muscle
24 Renal calix
25 Renal pyramid
26 Right lumbar lymph nodes
27 Paracolic lymph nodes
28 Inferior pancreatic-duodenal lymph nodes

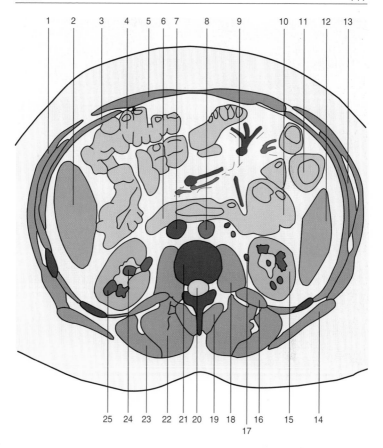

29 Superior mesenteric lymph nodes
30 Intermediate lumbar lymph nodes
31 Left lumbar lymph nodes
32 Juxtaintestinal lymph nodes

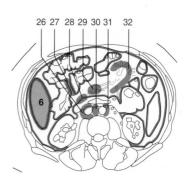

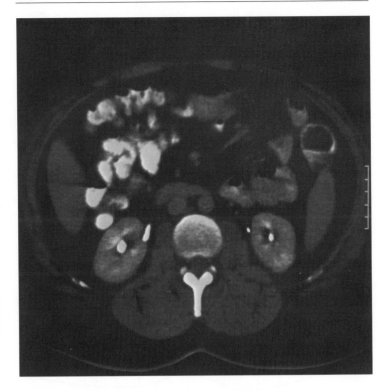

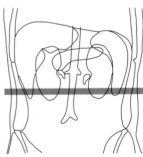

1 External oblique muscle
2 Liver
3 Transverse colon
4 Inferior vena cava
5 Duodenum
6 Abdominal aorta
7 Rectus abdominis muscle

8 Jejunal arteries and veins
9 Jejunum
10 Descending colon
11 Spleen
12 Internal oblique muscle
13 Transversus abdominis muscle
14 Left kidney
15 Quadratus lumborum muscle
16 Ureter
17 Psoas muscle
18 Lumbar vertebra 2
19 Spinal canal
20 Spinalis muscle
21 Longissimus thoracis muscle
22 Iliocostalis lumborum muscle
23 Renal calix
24 Renal pyramid
25 Latissimus dorsi muscle
26 Paracolic lymph nodes
27 Right lumbar lymph nodes
28 Intermediate lumbar lymph nodes

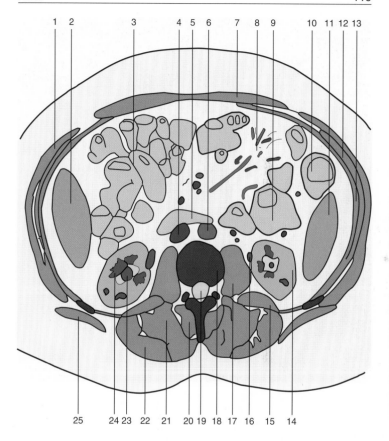

29 Superior mesenteric lymph nodes
30 Juxtaintestinal lymph nodes
31 Left lumbar lymph nodes

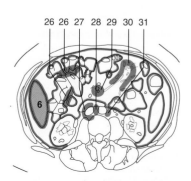

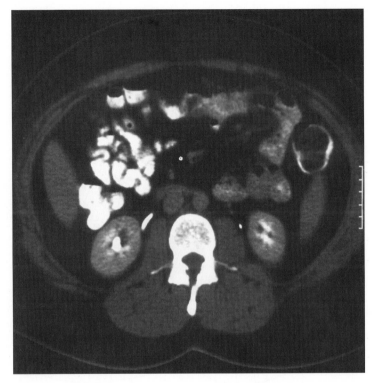

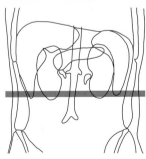

1 Liver
2 Ascending colon
3 Ileum
4 Transverse colon
5 Inferior vena cava
6 Duodenum
7 Abdominal aorta

8 Rectus abdominis muscle
9 Jejunal arteries and veins
10 Jejunum
11 Descending colon
12 Internal oblique muscle
13 External oblique muscle
14 Transversus abdominis muscle
15 Spleen
16 Left kidney
17 Iliocostalis lumborum muscle
18 Quadratus lumborum muscle
19 Longissimus thoracis muscle
20 Spinalis muscle
21 Spinal canal
22 Lumbar vertebra 3
23 Psoas muscle
24 Ureter
25 Renal calix
26 Renal pyramid
27 Latissimus dorsi muscle
28 Paracolic lymph nodes

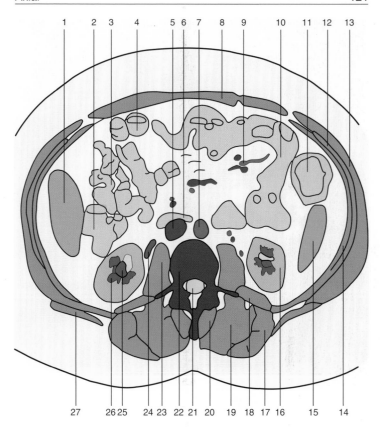

29 Lumbar lymph nodes
30 Intestinal lymph nodes
31 Intermediate lumbar lymph nodes
32 Left lumbar lymph nodes
33 Juxtaintestinal lymph nodes

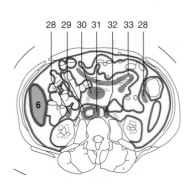

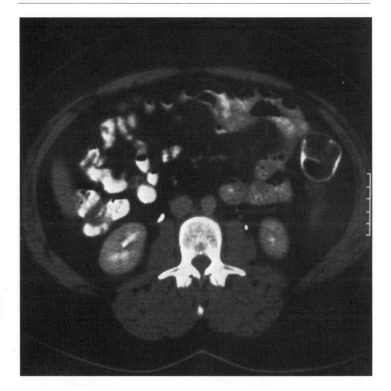

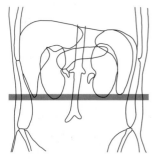

8 Jejunum
9 Descending colon
10 Internal oblique muscle
11 External oblique muscle
12 Transversus abdominis muscle
13 Spleen
14 Left kidney
15 Renal calix
16 Longissimus thoracis muscle
17 Spinalis muscle
18 Spinal canal
19 Lumbar vertebra 3
20 Psoas muscle
21 Iliocostalis lumborum muscle
22 Renal pyramid
23 Hepatic flexure of colon
24 Latissimus dorsi muscle
25 Paracolic lymph nodes
26 Juxtaintestinal lymph nodes
27 Lumbar lymph nodes
28 Intestinal lymph nodes

1 Liver
2 Ileum
3 Ureter
4 Inferior vena cava
5 Abdominal aorta
6 Rectus abdominis muscle
7 Jejunal arteries and veins

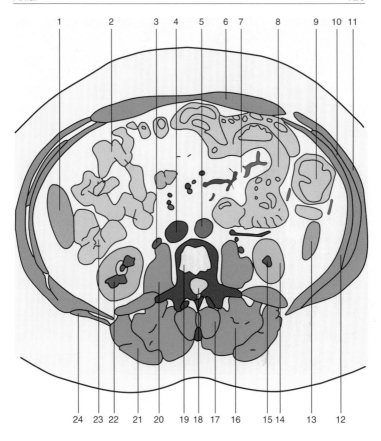

29 Intermediate lumbar lymph nodes
30 Left lumbar lymph nodes

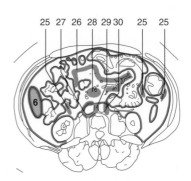

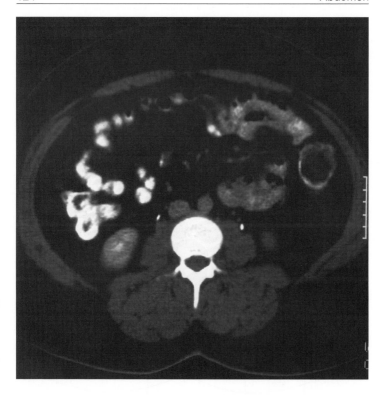

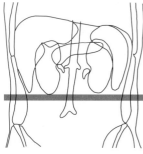

1 Liver
2 Right kidney
3 Right colic artery
4 Ureter
5 Inferior vena cava
6 Abdominal aorta
7 Inferior mesenteric artery

8 Jejunal arteries and veins
9 Rectus abdominis muscle
10 Jejunum
11 Descending colon
12 Internal oblique muscle
13 External oblique muscle
14 Transversus abdominis muscle
15 Quadratus lumborum muscle
16 Iliocostalis lumborum muscle
17 Longissimus thoracis muscle
18 Spinalis muscle
19 Spinal canal
20 Lumbar vertebra 3
21 Lumbar spinal nerve 1
22 Psoas muscle
23 Ascending colon
24 Paracolic lymph nodes
25 Juxtaintestinal lymph nodes
26 Right lumbar lymph nodes
27 Intermediate lumbar lymph nodes
28 Left lumbar lymph nodes

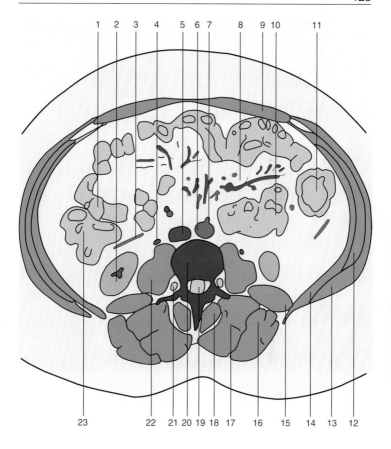

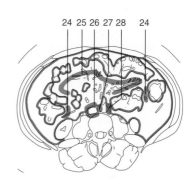

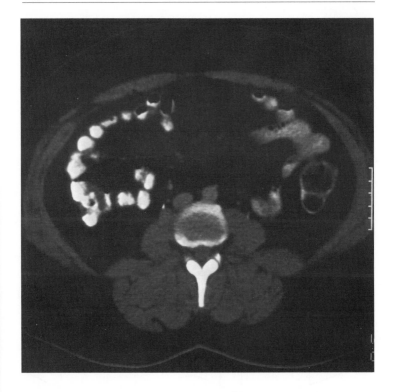

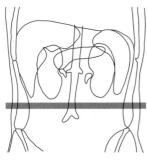

1 Ascending colon
2 Ileal arteries and veins
3 Rectus abdominis muscle
4 Ileum
5 Transverse colon
6 Inferior vena cava
7 Abdominal aorta

8 Inferior mesenteric artery
9 Jejunal arteries and veins
10 Jejunum
11 Descending colon
12 Quadratus lumborum muscle
13 Psoas muscle
14 Longissimus thoracis muscle
15 Spinalis muscle
16 Lumbar vertebra 3
17 Spinal canal
18 Spinal nerve root L2
19 Ureter
20 Iliocostalis lumborum muscle
21 Transversus abdominis muscle
22 Internal oblique muscle
23 External oblique muscle
24 Paracolic lymph nodes
25 Juxtaintestinal lymph nodes
26 Right lumbar lymph nodes
27 Intermediate lumbar lymph nodes
28 Inferior mesenteric lymph nodes

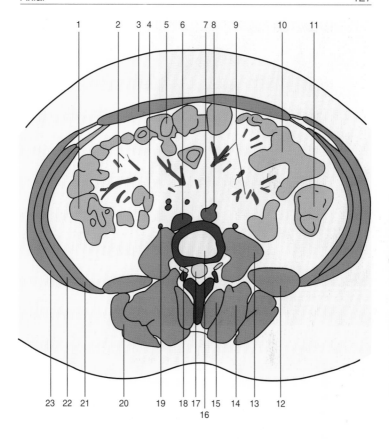

29 Left lumbar lymph nodes

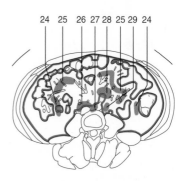

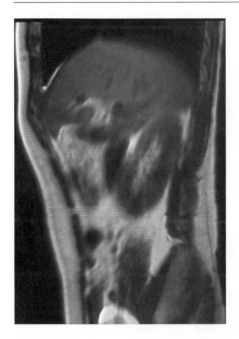

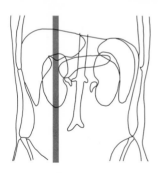

1 Right lung
2 Liver
3 Diaphragm
4 Rib 7
5 Round ligament of liver
6 Gall bladder
7 Ampulla of duodenum
8 Duodenum (descending part)
9 Transverse colon
10 Rectus abdominis muscle
11 Tendinous intersection
12 Ileal arteries and veins
13 Psoas muscle
14 External iliac artery
15 External iliac vein
16 Latissimus dorsi muscle
17 Rib 9
18 Portal vein
19 Diaphragm (lumbar part)
20 Parapelvic adipose tissue
21 Right kidney
22 Iliocostalis lumborum muscle
23 Quadratus lumborum muscle
24 Ilium

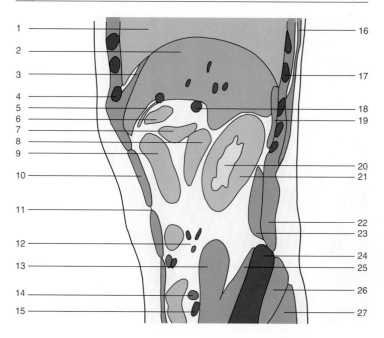

1
2
3
4
5
6
7
8
9
10
11
12
13
14
15

16
17
18
19
20
21
22
23
24
25
26
27

25 Iliacus muscle
26 Gluteus medius muscle
27 Gluteus maximus muscle
28 Paracolic lymph nodes
29 Mesenteric lymph nodes
30 External iliac lymph nodes

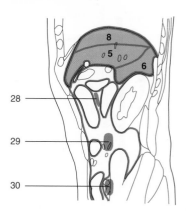

28
29
30

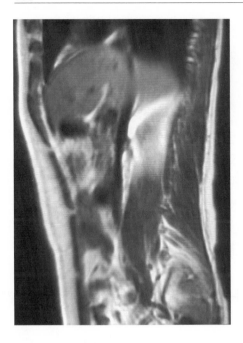

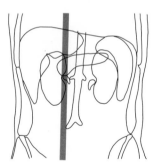

1 Right ventricle
2 Right lung
3 Diaphragm
4 Rib 7
5 Liver
6 Fissure for round ligament
7 Proper hepatic artery
8 Antrum
9 Duodenum (descending part)
10 Transverse colon
11 Rectus abdominis muscle
12 Tendinous intersection
13 Jejunum
14 Right common iliac artery
15 Right external iliac artery
16 Ileum
17 Right atrium
18 Longissimus thoracis muscle
19 Inferior vena cava
20 Portal vein
21 Right renal artery
22 Diaphragm (lumbar part)
23 Iliocostalis lumborum muscle
24 Psoas muscle

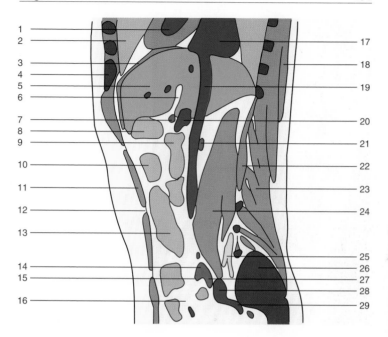

25 Lumbar plexus
26 Ilium
27 Right internal iliac artery
28 Right common iliac artery
29 Right internal iliac vein
30 Hepatic lymph nodes
31 Gastroomental lymph nodes
32 Postcaval lymph nodes
33 Common iliac lymph nodes

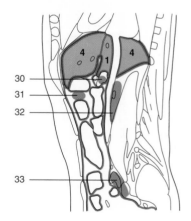

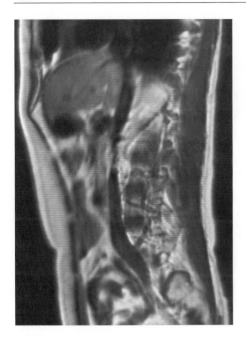

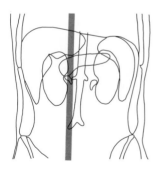

1 Sternum
2 Right lung
3 Right ventricle
4 Liver (right lobe)
5 Sternum (xyphoid process)
6 Proper hepatic artery
7 Pancreas
8 Stomach
9 Duodenum (horizontal part)
10 Jejunal arteries and veins
11 Transverse colon
12 Rectus abdominis muscle
13 Jejunum
14 Tendinous insertion
15 Ileal arteries and veins
16 Right internal iliac artery
17 Trapezius muscle
18 Right atrial appendage
19 Inferior vena cava
20 Liver (caudate lobe)
21 Ascending lumbar vein
22 Splenic vein
23 Right renal artery
24 Longissimus thoracis muscle

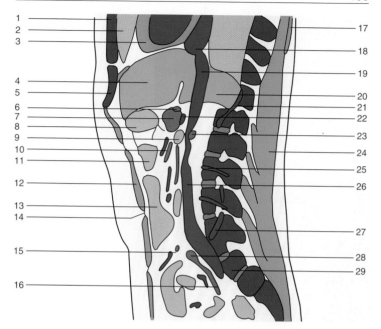

1
2
3
4
5
6
7
8
9
10
11
12
13
14
15
16

17
18
19
20
21
22
23
24
25
26
27
28
29

25 Lumbar vein
26 Inferior vena cava
27 Ascending lumbar vein
28 Right common iliac artery
29 Sacrum
30 Pancreatic lymph nodes
31 Gastroomental lymph nodes
32 Superior mesenteric lymph nodes
33 Intermediate lumbar lymph nodes
34 Common iliac lymph nodes
35 Internal iliac lymph nodes
36 Juxtaintestinal lymph nodes

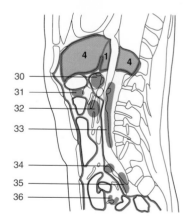

30
31
32
33
34
35
36

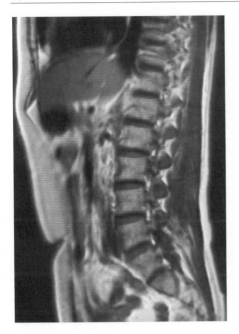

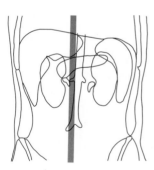

1 Right atrium
2 Right ventricle
3 Sternum
4 Liver
5 Hepatic vein
6 Fissure for round ligament
7 Hepatic artery
8 Pancreas
9 Stomach
10 Splenic vein
11 Jejunal artery
12 Gastroomental artery
13 Transverse colon
14 Jejunum
15 Umbilicus
16 Rectus abdominis muscle
17 Tendinous intersection
18 Ileum
19 Trapezius muscle
20 Right lung
21 Duodenum (horizontal part)
22 Left renal artery
23 Spinal nerve root L1
24 Superior mesenteric vein

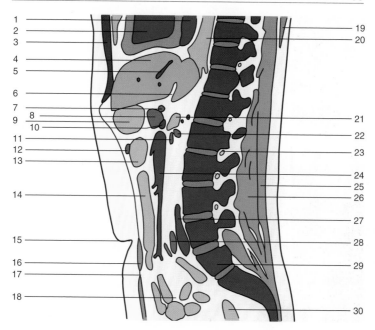

25 Longissimus thoracis muscle
26 Spinalis muscle
27 Left common iliac vein
28 Left common iliac artery
29 Lumbar vertebra 5
30 Rectum
31 Prepericardial lymph nodes
32 Pancreatic lymph nodes
33 Gastroomental lymph nodes
34 Superior mesenteric lymph nodes
35 External iliac lymph nodes
36 Mesenteric lymph nodes

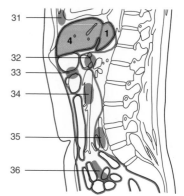

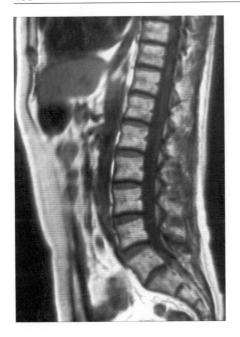

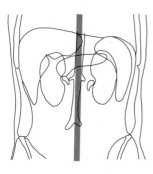

1 Sternum
2 Left ventricle
3 Right ventricle
4 Rib 7
5 Liver
6 Diaphragm
7 Rectus abdominis muscle
8 Pancreas
9 Splenic vein
10 Stomach
11 Superior mesenteric artery
12 Left renal vein
13 Gastroomental lymph artery
14 Transverse colon
15 Linea alba
16 Superior mesenteric artery
17 Jejunum
18 Left iliac vein
19 Left iliac artery
20 Ileal arteries and veins
21 Ileum
22 Left lung
23 Esophagus
24 Spinal cord

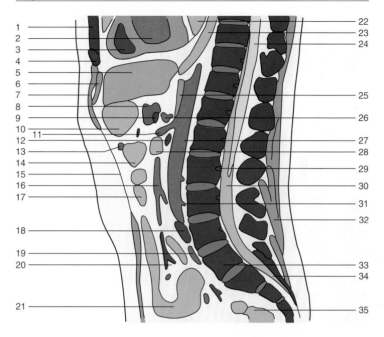

25 Diaphragm (lumbar part)
26 Celiac trunk
27 Abdominal aorta
28 Duodenum (horizontal part)
29 Basivertebral vein (nutrient foramen)
30 Spinal canal
31 Lumbar artery
32 Spinalis muscle
33 Lumbar vertebra 5
34 Sacral canal
35 Rectum
36 Superior phrenic lymph nodes
37 Inferior phrenic lymph nodes
38 Prevertebral lymph nodes
39 Pancreatic lymph nodes
40 Superior mesenteric lymph nodes
41 Gastroomental lymph nodes
42 Intestinal lymph nodes
43 Common iliac lymph nodes
44 Juxtaintestinal lymph nodes

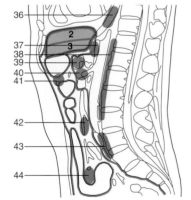

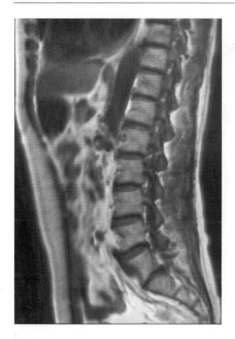

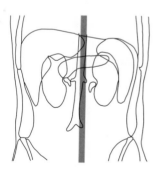

1 Left lung
2 Right ventricle
3 Left ventricle
4 Rib 7
5 Esophagus (abdominal part)
6 Liver
7 Splenic artery
8 Pancreas
9 Stomach
10 Duodenum (inferior part)
11 Transverse colon
12 Jejunal arteries and veins
13 Rectus abdominis muscle
14 Jejunum
15 Tendinous intersection
16 Ileal arteries and veins
17 Left common iliac artery
18 Left common iliac vein
19 Ileum
20 Abdominal aorta
21 Splenic vein
22 Left renal artery and vein
23 Spinal nerve root L2
24 Spinalis muscle

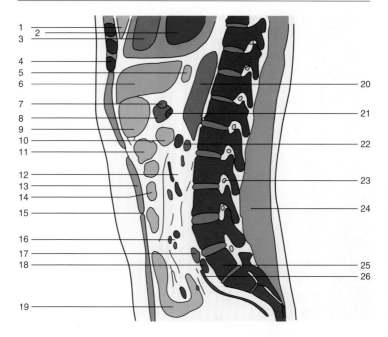

25 Lumbar vertebra 5
26 Middle sacral vein
27 Superior phrenic lymph nodes
28 Parasternal lymph nodes
29 Inferior phrenic lymph nodes
30 Pancreatic lymph nodes
31 Left lumbar lymph nodes
32 Gastroomental lymph nodes
33 Superior mesenteric lymph nodes
34 Intestinal lymph nodes
35 Common iliac lymph nodes
36 Juxtaintestinal lymph nodes
37 Presacral lymph nodes

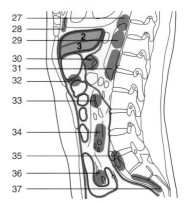

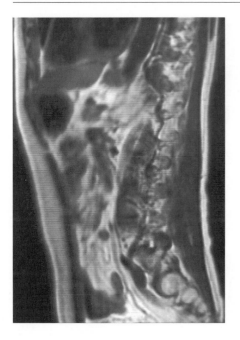

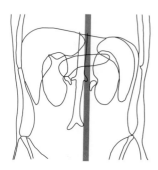

1 Left lung
2 Left ventricle
3 Right ventricle
4 Rib 5
5 Liver
6 Splenic artery
7 Pancreas
8 Stomach
9 Duodenum (inferior part)
10 Gastroepiploic artery
11 Transverse colon
12 Jejunal arteries and veins
13 Jejunum
14 Tendinous intersection
15 Rectus abdominis muscle
16 Ileal arteries and veins
17 Left common iliac artery
18 Left common iliac vein
19 Ileum
20 Trapezius muscle
21 Descending aorta
22 Hemiazygos vein
23 Esophagus (abdominal part)
24 Spinalis muscle

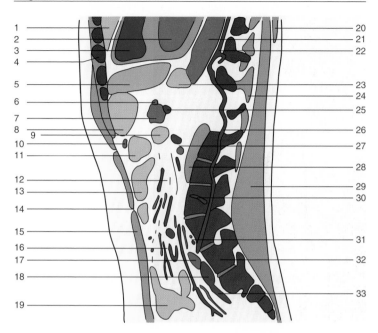

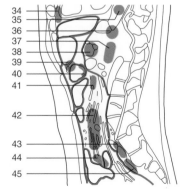

25 Splenic vein
26 Ascending lumbar vein
27 Left renal artery and vein
28 Psoas muscle
29 Longissimus thoracis muscle
30 Lumbar vein
31 Lumbar artery and vein
32 Lumbar vertebra 5
33 Left internal iliac vein
34 Parasternal lymph nodes
35 Superior phrenic lymph nodes
36 Inferior phrenic lymph nodes
37 Left lumbar lymph nodes
38 Pancreatic lymph nodes
39 Gastroomental lymph nodes
40 Paracolic lymph nodes
41 Superior mesenteric lymph nodes
42 Intestinal lymph nodes
43 Common iliac lymph nodes
44 Juxtaintestinal lymph nodes
45 Internal iliac lymph nodes

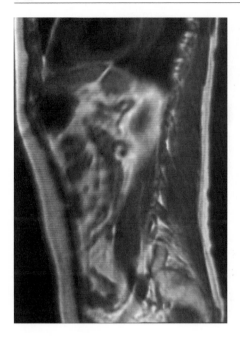

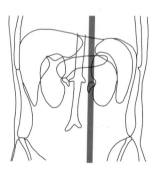

1 Left ventricle
2 Papillary muscle
3 Rib 6
4 Liver
5 Stomach
6 Splenic artery and vein
7 Pancreas
8 Duodenum (inferior part)
9 Transverse colon
10 Jejunal arteries and veins
11 Jejunum
12 Rectus abdominis muscle
13 Ileal arteries and veins
14 Left external iliac artery
15 Ileum
16 Left external iliac vein
17 Trapezius muscle
18 Descending aorta
19 Rib 10
20 Left lung
21 Esophagus
22 Left adrenal gland
23 Left kidney
24 Longissimus thoracis muscle

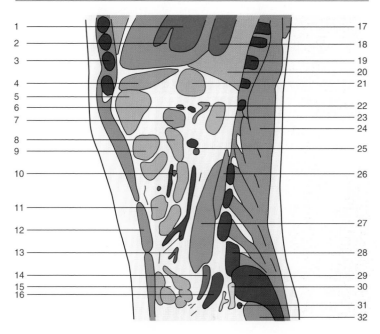

1
2
3
4
5
6
7
8
9
10
11
12
13
14
15
16

17
18
19
20
21
22
23
24
25
26
27
28
29
30
31
32

25 Left renal artery and vein
26 Psoas minor muscle
27 Psoas major muscle
28 Sacrum (superior articular process)
29 Sacrum
30 Sacral plexus
31 Superior gluteal vein
32 Piriformis muscle
33 Pancreatic lymph nodes
34 Gastroomental lymph nodes
35 Paracolic lymph nodes
36 Inferior duodenal lymph nodes
37 Intestinal lymph nodes
38 External iliac lymph nodes

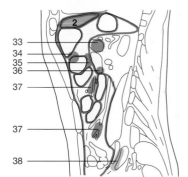

33
34
35
36
37

37

38

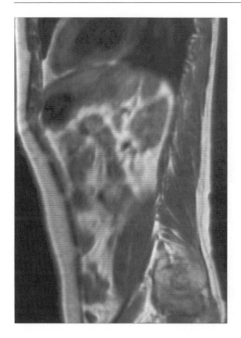

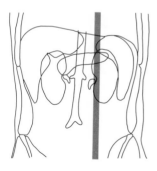

1 Left ventricle
2 Rib 5
3 Diaphragm
4 Stomach
5 Pancreas
6 Duodenum (inferior part)
7 Transverse colon
8 Jejunum
9 Jejunal and Ileal arteries and veins
10 Rectus abdominis muscle
11 Tendinous intersection
12 Psoas major muscle
13 Ileum
14 Left external iliac artery
15 Left external iliac vein
16 Left lung
17 Latissimus dorsi muscle
18 Spleen
19 Rib 12
20 Splenic vein
21 Left kidney
22 Quadratus lumborum muscle
23 Left renal artery and vein
24 Longissimus thoracis muscle

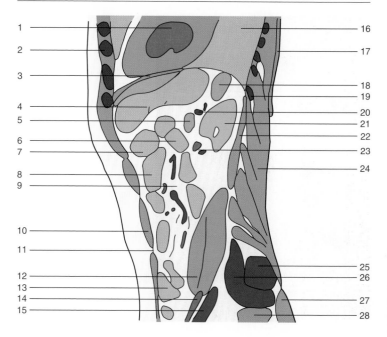

1
2
3
4
5
6
7
8
9
10
11
12
13
14
15

16
17
18
19
20
21
22
23
24
25
26
27
28

25 Ilium
26 Sacral ala
27 Gluteus maximus muscle
28 Piriformis muscle
29 Intercostal lymph nodes
30 Gastroomental lymph nodes
31 Pancreatic lymph nodes
32 Intestinal lymph nodes
33 External iliac lymph nodes

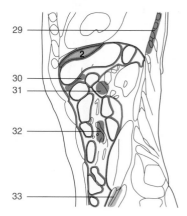

29
30
31
32
33

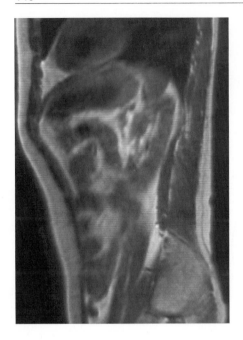

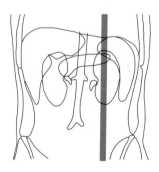

1 Left ventricle
2 Rib 4
3 Diaphragm
4 Liver
5 Splenic vein
6 Pancreas
7 Duodenojejunal flexure
8 Transverse colon
9 Rectus abdominis muscle
10 Jejunum
11 Tendinous intersection
12 Ileal artery and vein
13 Left lung
14 Latissimus dorsi muscle
15 Spleen
16 Left kidney
17 Renal vein
18 Renal artery
19 Parapelvic adipose tissue
20 Quadratus lumborum muscle
21 Iliocostalis lumborum muscle
22 Longissimus thoracis muscle
23 Psoas major muscle
24 Psoas minor muscle

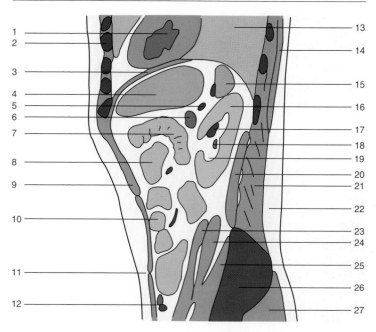

25 Iliacus muscle
26 Ilium
27 Gluteus maximus muscle
28 Intercostal lymph nodes
29 Pancreatic lymph nodes
30 Gastroomental lymph nodes
31 Juxtaintestinal lymph nodes
32 External iliac lymph nodes

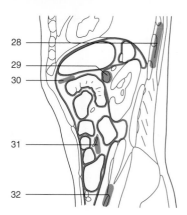

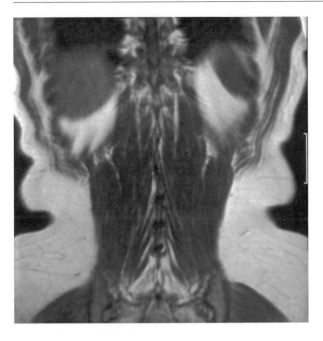

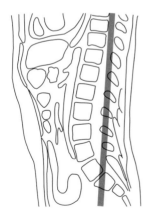

1 Right lung
2 Serratus anterior muscle
3 Liver
4 Latissimus dorsi muscle
5 Lumbar trigone (Petit's)
6 Multifidus muscles
7 Ilium
8 Sacral ala
9 Spinal cord
10 Spinal canal
11 Spleen
12 Quadratus lumborum muscle
13 Longissimus thoracis muscle
14 Iliocostalis lumborum muscle
15 Sacral vertebra 1
16 Gluteus maximus muscle
17 Intercostal lymph nodes

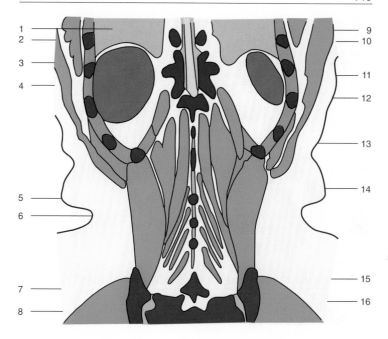

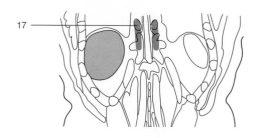

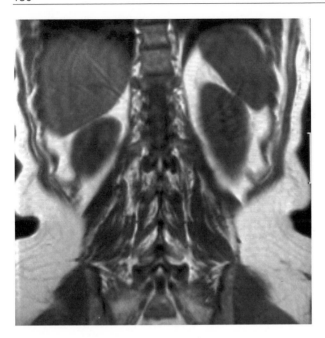

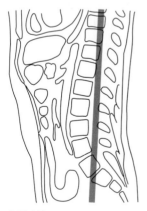

1 Right lung
2 Serratus anterior muscle
3 Posterior intercostal artery
4 Liver
5 Latissimus dorsi muscle
6 Transversus abdominis muscle

7 Inferior posterior serratus anterior
  muscle
8 Internal oblique muscle
9 Quadratus lumborum muscle
10 Iliocostalis lumborum muscle
11 Longissimus thoracis muscle
12 Ilium
13 Sacral ala
14 Sacroiliac joint
15 Descending aorta
16 Hemiazygos vein
17 Diaphragm
18 Spleen
19 Rib 12
20 Rib 11
21 Spinal canal
22 Left kidney
23 Multifidus muscles
24 Sacral canal
25 Gluteus maximus muscle
26 Superior phrenic lymph nodes

1
2
3
4
5
6
7
8
9
10
11
12
13
14

15
16
17
18
19
20
21
22
23
24
25

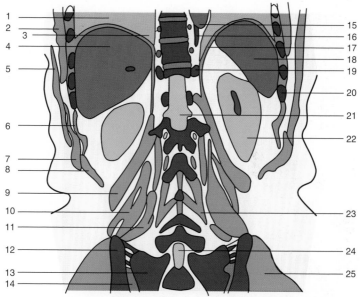

26

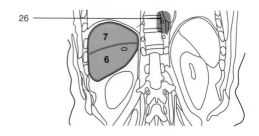

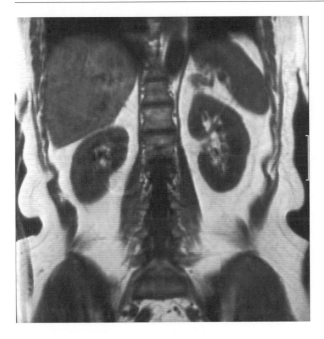

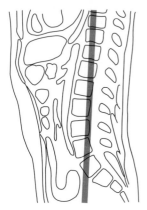

1 Azygos vein
2 Right lung
3 Diaphragm
4 Inferior vena cava
5 Liver
6 Left adrenal gland

7 Diaphragm (lumbar part)
8 Major renal calyces
9 Right kidney
10 External oblique muscle
11 Internal oblique muscle
12 Transversus abdominis muscle
13 Ilium
14 Sacrum
15 Iliacus muscle
16 Superior gluteal artery
17 Internal iliac artery
18 Esophagus
19 Serratus anterior muscle
20 Abdominal aorta
21 Spleen
22 Splenic vein
23 Splenic artery
24 Latissimus dorsi muscle
25 Lumbar vertebra 1
26 Minor renal calyces
27 Lumbar artery
28 Spinal canal
29 Psoas muscle
30 Multifidus muscles

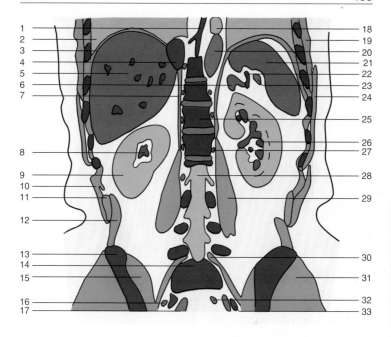

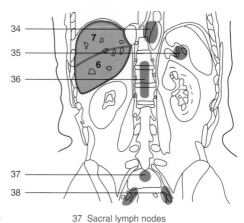

31 Gluteus maximus muscle
32 Superior rectal artery
33 Internal iliac vein
34 Superior phrenic lymph nodes
35 Splenic lymph nodes
36 Prevertebral lymph nodes

37 Sacral lymph nodes
38 Internal iliac lymph nodes

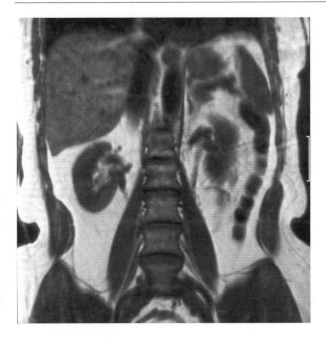

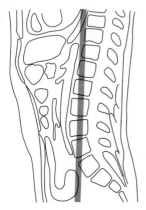

1 Right atrium
2 Right lung
3 Serratus anterior muscle
4 Inferior vena cava
5 Abdominal aorta
6 Liver

7 Right adrenal gland
8 Diaphragm (lumbar part)
9 Renal artery
10 Renal vein
11 Renal calyx
12 Right kidney
13 External oblique muscle
14 Internal oblique muscle
15 Transversus abdominis muscle
16 Ilium
17 Gluteus maximus muscle
18 Iliacus muscle
19 Left ventricle
20 Diaphragm
21 Esophagus
22 Stomach
23 Spleen
24 Splenic vein
25 Left gastric artery
26 Splenic artery
27 Pancreas
28 Descending colon
29 Renal pelvis
30 Latissimus dorsi muscle

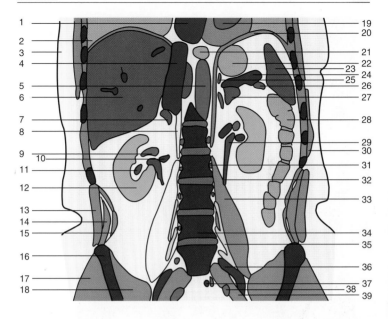

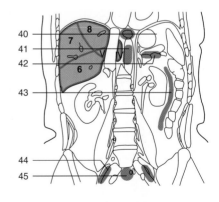

31 Lumbar artery
32 Ureter
33 Psoas muscle
34 Lumbar vertebra 5
35 Lumbar plexus
36 Internal iliac vein
37 Median sacral artery and vein
38 Internal iliac artery
39 Piriformis muscle

40 Superior phrenic lymph nodes
41 Inferior phrenic lymph nodes
42 Pancreatic lymph nodes
43 Paracolic lymph nodes
44 Internal iliac lymph nodes
45 Sacral lymph nodes

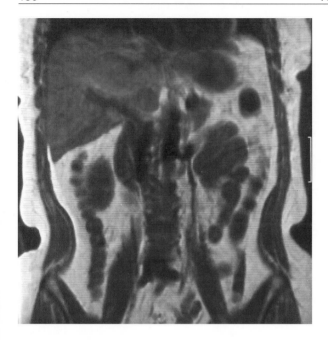

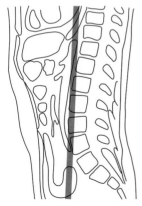

1 Left ventricle
2 Right ventricle
3 Coronary sinus
4 Liver
5 Pancreas (head)
6 Portal vein

7 Superior mesenteric artery
8 Inferior vena cava
9 Right renal artery
10 Right kidney
11 Ascending colon
12 External oblique muscle
13 Internal oblique muscle
14 Transversus abdominis muscle
15 Iliacus muscle
16 Ileal veins
17 Gluteus medius muscle
18 Left lung
19 Serratus anterior muscle
20 Liver (left lobe)
21 Stomach
22 Splenic flexure of colon
23 Splenic artery and vein
24 Pancreas (body)
25 Abdominal aorta
26 Left renal vein
27 Left kidney
28 Ureter
29 Lumbar artery
30 Lumbar vertebra 4

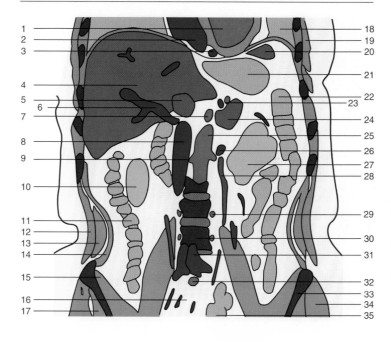

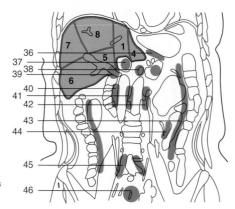

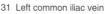

31 Left common iliac vein
32 Right internal iliac artery
33 Ilium
34 Gluteus maximus muscle
35 Ileum
36 Gastroomental lymph nodes
37 Pancreatic lymph nodes
38 Hepatic lymph nodes
39 Superior mesenteric lymph
   nodes
40 Right lumbar lymph nodes
   (lateral caval)
41 Intermediate lumbar lymph
   nodes

42 Left lumbar lymph nodes
43 Paracolic lymph nodes
44 Juxtaintestinal lymph nodes
45 Common iliac lymph nodes
46 Intestinal lymph nodes

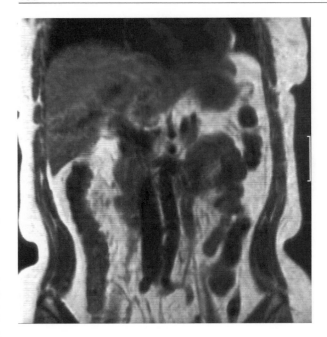

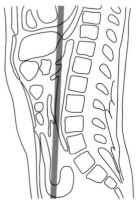

1 Left ventricle
2 Right ventricle
3 Right coronary artery
4 Liver
5 Celiac trunk
6 Portal vein

7 Common hepatic artery
8 Pancreas
9 Duodenum
10 Superior mesenteric artery
11 Jejunum
12 Ascending colon
13 Right colic veins
14 Inferior vena cava
15 External oblique muscle
16 Superior mesenteric vein
17 Internal oblique muscle
18 Transversus abdominis muscle
19 Right common iliac vein
20 Iliacus muscle
21 Gluteus maximus muscle
22 Left lung
23 Serratus anterior muscle
24 Diaphragm
25 Stomach
26 Splenic artery
27 Splenic vein
28 Pancreas (body)
29 Descending colon
30 Left renal artery

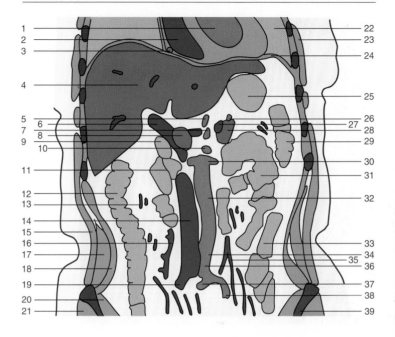

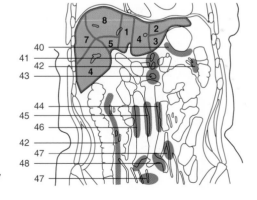

31 Jejunum
32 Abdominal aorta
33 Descending colon
34 Left common iliac artery
35 Ileal veins
36 Internal iliac artery
37 Middle rectal artery
38 Internal pudendal artery
39 Ilium
40 Gastroomental lymph nodes
41 Celiac lymph nodes
42 Paracolic lymph nodes

43 Superior mesenteric lymph nodes
44 Left lumbar lymph nodes
45 Intermediate lumbar lymph nodes
46 Lumbar lateral caval lymph nodes
47 Mesenteric lymph nodes
48 Common iliac lymph nodes

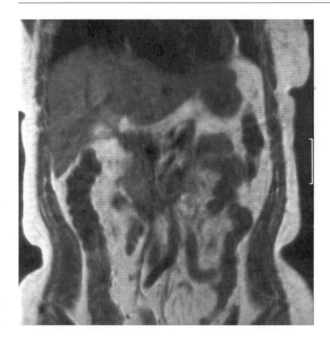

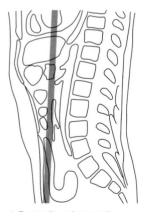

1 Pectoralis major muscle
2 Right ventricle
3 Right coronary artery
4 Liver
5 Pancreas (head)
6 Superior mesenteric vein

7   Inferior mesenteric artery
8   Hepatic flexure of colon
9   Abdominal aorta
10 Ascending colon
11 Inferior mesenteric vein
12 External oblique muscle
13 Internal oblique muscle
14 Transversus abdominis muscle
15 Ilium
16 Left lung
17 Left ventricle
18 Serratus anterior muscle
19 Diaphragm
20 Stomach
21 Celiac trunk
22 Splenic flexure of colon
23 Common hepatic artery
24 Superior mesenteric artery
25 Pancreas (tail)
26 Jejunum
27 Jejunal veins
28 Descending colon
29 Left common iliac artery
30 Iliac veins

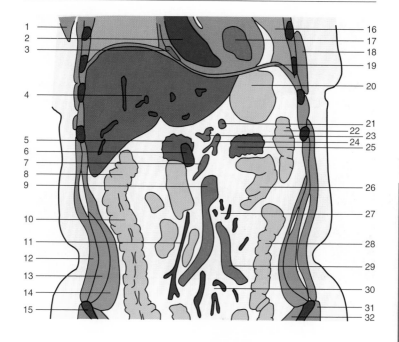

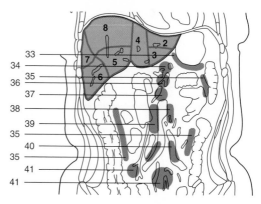

31 Gluteus maximus muscle
32 Iliacus muscle
33 Gastroomental lymph nodes
34 Celiac lymph nodes
35 Paracolic lymph nodes
36 Superior mesenteric lymph nodes

37 Inferior mesenteric lymph nodes
38 Left lumbar lymph nodes
39 Right lumbar lymph nodes (precaval)
40 Common iliac lymph nodes
41 Intestinal lymph nodes

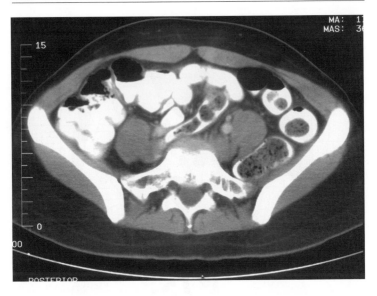

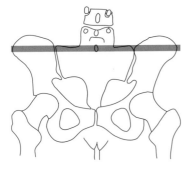

1 Rectus abdominis muscle
2 Internal oblique muscle
3 External oblique muscle
4 Transverse colon
5 Common iliac artery and vein
6 Ileum
7 Rectus abdominis muscle
8 Ureter
9 Transverse colon
10 Gluteus medius muscle
11 Iliacus muscle
12 Descending colon
13 Longissimus thoracis muscle
14 Spinalis muscle
15 Spinal nerve S1
16 Spinal canal
17 Intervertebral disk, promontory
18 Sacrum
19 Psoas muscle

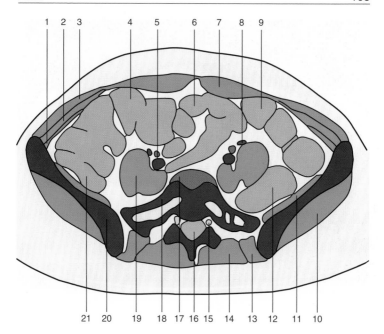

20 Ilium
21 Ascending colon
22 Paracolic lymph nodes
23 Intermediate common iliac lymph nodes
24 Common iliac lymph nodes of promontory
25 Juxtaintestinal lymph nodes
26 Medial common iliac lymph nodes
27 Lateral common iliac lymph nodes

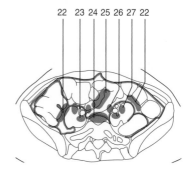

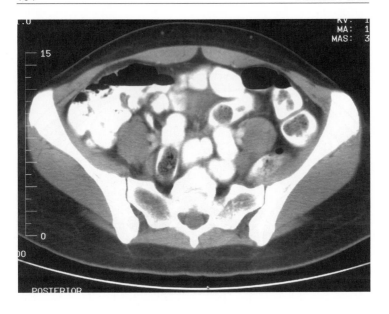

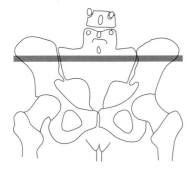

1 Iliacus muscle
2 Ascending colon
3 Ureter
4 Inferior epigastric artery
5 Ileum
6 Urinary bladder
7 Rectus abdominis muscle
8 Common iliac artery and vein
9 Psoas muscle
10 Transverse colon
11 Internal oblique muscle
12 Rectus abdominis muscle
13 External oblique muscle
14 Ilium (ala)
15 Gluteus medius muscle
16 Gluteus maximus muscle
17 Descending colon
18 Jejunum
19 spinal canal

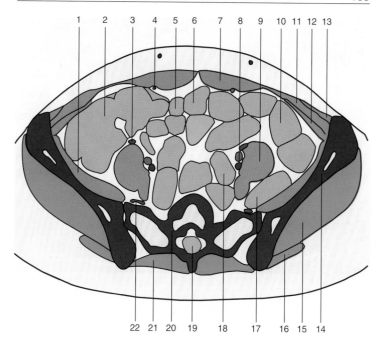

20 Sacrum
21 Spinalis muscle
22 Sacral plexus
23 Paracolic lymph nodes
24 Lateral common iliac lymph nodes
25 Medial common iliac lymph nodes
26 Juxtaintestinal lymph nodes
27 Common iliac lymph nodes of
   promontory
28 Intermediate common iliac lymph
   nodes

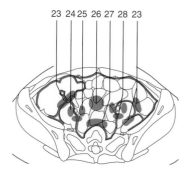

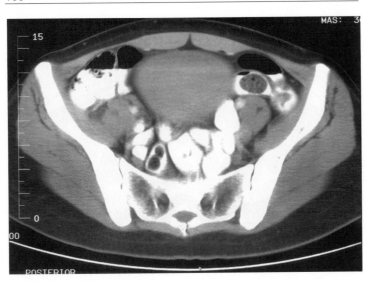

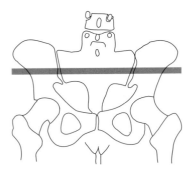

1 Internal oblique muscle
2 Transversus abdominis muscle
3 Ascending colon
4 Psoas muscle
5 Ureter
6 Inferior epigastric artery
7 Jejunum
8 Urinary bladder
9 Rectus abdominis muscle
10 External iliac artery and vein
11 Descending colon
12 Iliacus muscle
13 Ilium (ala)
14 Gluteus minimus muscle
15 Gluteus medius muscle
16 Gluteus maximus muscle
17 Sacroiliac joint
18 Spinalis muscle
19 Spinal canal

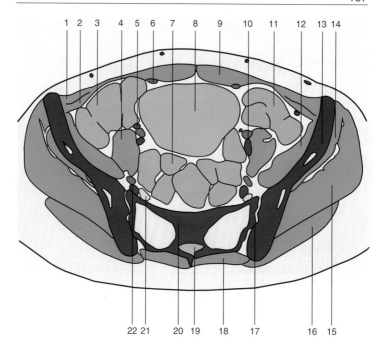

20 Sacrum
21 Sacral plexus
22 Internal iliac artery and vein
23 Paracolic lymph nodes
24 Superior gluteal lymph nodes
25 Medial external iliac lymph nodes
26 Juxtaintestinal lymph nodes
27 Sacral lymph nodes
28 Interiliac external iliac lymph nodes
29 Lateral external iliac lymph nodes

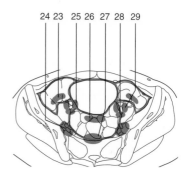

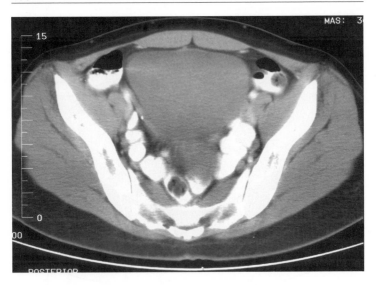

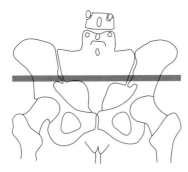

1 Tensor fasciae latae muscle
2 Transversus abdominis muscle
3 Internal oblique muscle
4 Cecum
5 External iliac artery and vein
6 Inferior epigastric artery
7 Round ligament of uterus
8 Urinary bladder
9 Rectus abdominis muscle
10 Psoas muscle
11 Descending colon
12 Iliacus muscle
13 Ilium (ala)
14 Sacroiliac joint
15 Sigmoid colon
16 Piriformis muscle
17 Uterus
18 Rectum
19 Sacral canal

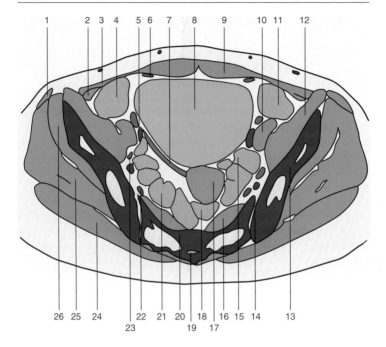

20 Sacrum
21 Ileum
22 Sacral plexus
23 Internal iliac artery and vein
24 Gluteus maximus muscle
25 Gluteus medius muscle
26 Gluteus minimus muscle
27 Lateral external iliac lymph nodes
28 Intermediate external iliac lymph nodes
29 Medial external iliac lymph nodes
30 Juxtaintestinal lymph nodes
31 Sacral lymph nodes
32 Pararectal lymph nodes
33 Paracolic lymph nodes
34 Superior gluteal lymph nodes

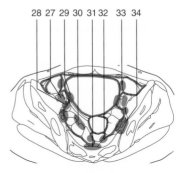

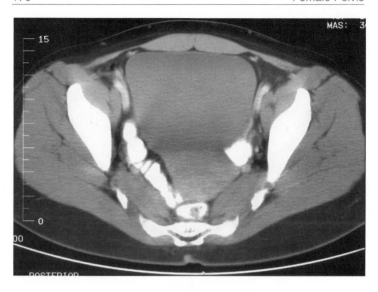

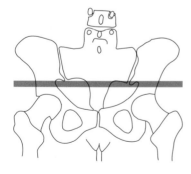

1 Tensor fasciae latae muscle
2 Sartorius muscle
3 Internal oblique muscle
4 External iliac artery and vein
5 Inferior epigastric artery and vein
6 Round ligament of uterus
7 Urinary bladder
8 Uterus
9 Rectus abdominis muscle
10 Ovary
11 Ilium (ala)
12 Iliopsoas muscle
13 Ovarian artery and vein
14 Internal iliac artery and vein
15 Sacrum
16 Rectum
17 Sacral canal
18 Piriformis muscle
19 Ileum

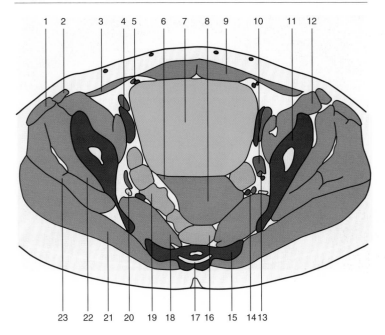

20 Sacral plexus
21 Gluteus maximus muscle
22 Gluteus minimus muscle
23 Gluteus medius muscle
24 Lateral external iliac lymph nodes
25 Intermediate external iliac lymph nodes
26 Parauterine lymph nodes
27 Sacral lymph nodes
28 Pararectal lymph nodes
29 Medial external iliac lymph nodes
30 Superior gluteal lymph nodes

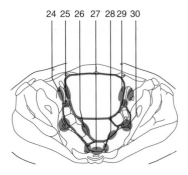

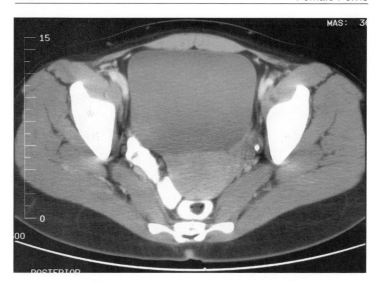

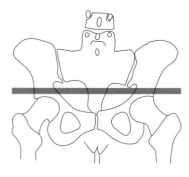

1 Tensor fasciae latae muscle
2 Sartorius muscle
3 Iliopsoas muscle
4 External iliac artery and vein
5 Superior vesical artery and vein
6 Rectus abdominis muscle
7 Urinary bladder
8 Uterus
9 Round ligament of uterus
10 Inferior epigastric artery and vein
11 Femoral nerve
12 Ilium (body)
13 Superior gluteal artery and vein
14 Ovary
15 Uterine artery and vein
16 Rectum
17 Sacral hiatus
18 Sacrum
19 Piriformis muscle

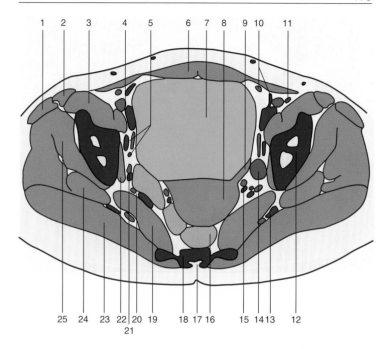

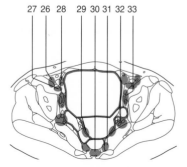

20 Inferior gluteal artery and vein
21 Internal iliac artery and vein
22 Internal obturator muscle
23 Gluteus maximus muscle
24 Gluteus medius muscle
25 Gluteus minimus muscle
26 Lateral external iliac lymph nodes
27 Intermediate external iliac lymph nodes
28 Medial external iliac lymph nodes
29 Parauterine lymph nodes
30 Sacral lymph nodes
31 Pararectal lymph nodes
32 Inferior gluteal lymph nodes
33 Lateral vesicular lymph nodes

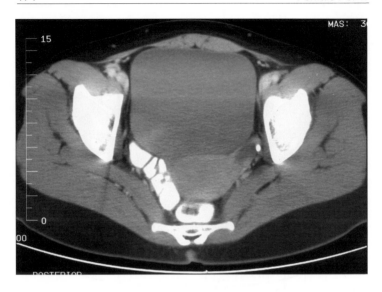

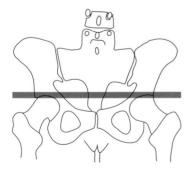

1 Tensor fasciae latae muscle
2 Sartorius muscle
3 Iliopsoas muscle
4 Deep circumflex iliac vein
5 Inferior epigastric artery and vein
6 Ureter
7 Internal oblique muscle
8 Urinary bladder
9 Uterus
10 Rectus abdominis muscle
11 Ovary
12 Corpus luteum
13 Superior vesical artery
14 External iliac artery and vein
15 Femoral nerve
16 Ilium (body)
17 Gluteus medius muscle
18 Gluteus minimus muscle
19 Gluteus maximus muscle

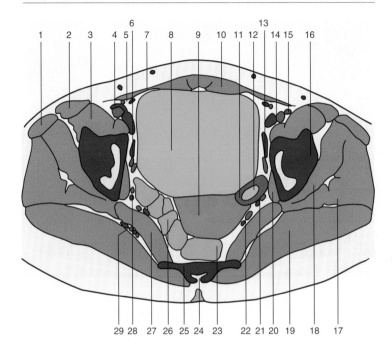

1 2 3 4 5 6 7 8 9 10 11 12 13 14 15 16

29 28 27 26 25 24 23 22 21 20 19 18 17

20 Internal obturator muscle
21 Ovarian artery and vein
22 Uterine artery and vein
23 Rectum
24 Sacral hiatus
25 Sacrum
26 Ileum
27 Piriformis muscle
28 Internal pudendal artery and vein
29 Inferior gluteal artery and vein
30 Lateral external iliac lymph nodes
31 Intermediate external iliac lymph nodes
32 Medial external iliac lymph nodes
33 Inferior gluteal lymph nodes
34 Postvesicular lymph nodes
35 Parauterine lymph nodes
36 Sacral lymph nodes
37 Pararectal lymph nodes
38 Lateral vesicular lymph nodes

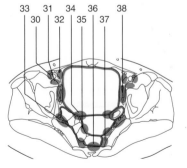

33 31 34 36 38
30 32 35 37

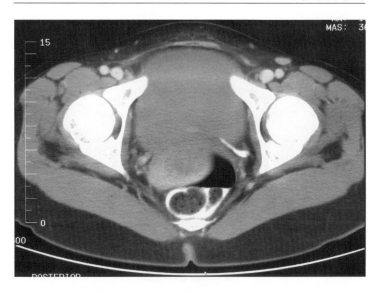

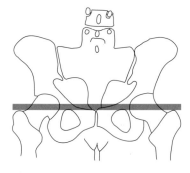

1 Tensor fasciae latae muscle
2 Sartorius muscle
3 Femoral nerve
4 External iliac artery and vein
5 Medial external iliac lymph node
6 Pubic bone
7 Urinary bladder
8 Rectus abdominis muscle
9 Uterus
10 Ureter
11 Internal oblique muscle
12 Obturator artery
13 Internal obturator muscle
14 Fovea of head of femur
15 Superficial inguinal lymph nodes
16 Iliopsoas muscle
17 Rectus femoris muscle
18 Head of femur
19 Inferior gluteal artery and vein

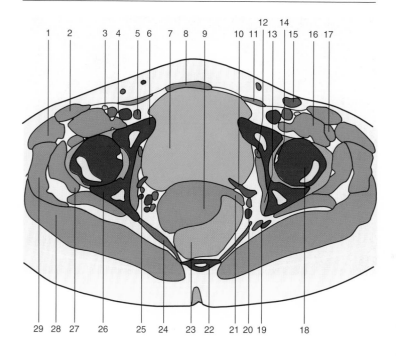

20 Inferior vesical artery and vein
21 Fallopian tube
22 Coccyx
23 Rectum
24 Sacrospinal ligament
25 Internal pudendal artery and vein
26 Ischium
27 Gluteus minimus muscle
28 Gluteus maximus muscle
29 Gluteus medius muscle
30 Lateral external iliac lymph nodes
31 Intermediate external iliac lymph nodes
32 Medial external iliac lymph nodes
33 Inferior gluteal lymph nodes
34 Parauterine lymph nodes
35 Pararectal lymph nodes
36 Postvesicular lymph nodes
37 Lateral vesicular lymph nodes
38 Superficial inguinal lymph nodes

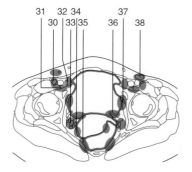

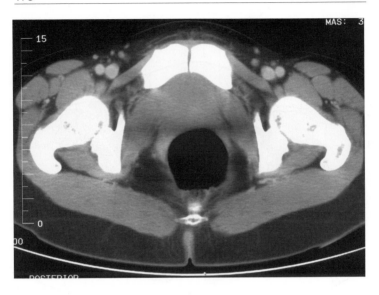

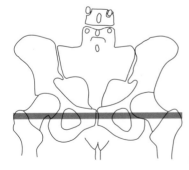

1 Tensor fasciae latae muscle
2 Lateral femoral circumflex artery
  (ascending branch)
3 Sartorius muscle
4 Iliopsoas muscle
5 Superficial iliac circumflex artery and vein
6 Obturator artery and vein
7 Pectineus muscle
8 Internal obturator muscle
9 Pubic bone (superior ramus)
10 Urinary bladder
11 Pubic symphysis
12 Uterus (cervix)
13 Levator ani muscle
14 External obturator muscle
15 Superficial epigastric artery and vein
16 Femoral artery and vein
17 Femoral nerve
18 Rectus femoris muscle

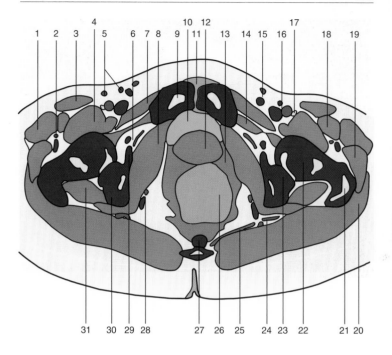

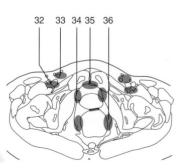

19 Gluteus medius muscle
20 Gluteus maximus muscle
21 Greater trochanter
22 Head of femur
23 Acetabulum
24 Inferior gluteal artery and vein
25 Sacrospinal ligament
26 Rectum
27 Coccyx
28 Internal pudendal artery and vein
29 Pubic bone
30 Ischium
31 Superior and inferior gemellus muscles
32 Deep inguinal lymph nodes
33 Superficial inguinal lymph nodes
34 Paravaginal lymph nodes
35 Prevesicular lymph nodes
36 Pararectal lymph nodes

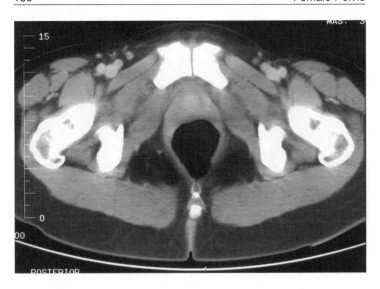

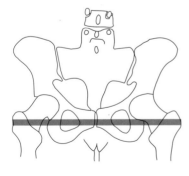

1 Gluteal fascia
2 Tensor fasciae latae muscle
3 Vastus lateralis muscle
4 Rectus femoris muscle
5 Sartorius muscle
6 Superficial iliac circumflex vein
7 Femoral artery and vein
8 Superficial epigastric artery and vein
9 Obturator artery and vein
10 Bulbocavernosus muscle
11 Vagina
12 Urethra
13 Ischiocavernosus muscle
14 Internal obturator muscle
15 External obturator muscle
16 Pectineus muscle
17 Great saphenous vein
18 Femoral nerve
19 Iliopsoas muscle

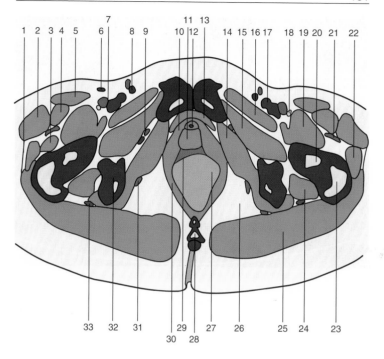

20 Neck of femur
21 Lateral femoral circumflex artery
22 Gluteus medius muscle
23 Greater trochanter
24 Quadratus femoris muscle
25 Gluteus maximus muscle
26 Ischiorectal fossa
27 Rectum
28 Coccyx
29 Central tendon of perineum
30 Levator ani muscle
31 Internal pudendal artery
32 Ischium
33 Sciatic nerve
34 Deep inguinal lymph nodes
35 Superficial inguinal lymph nodes
36 Paravaginal lymph nodes
37 Prevesicular lymph nodes
38 Pararectal lymph nodes

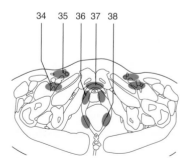

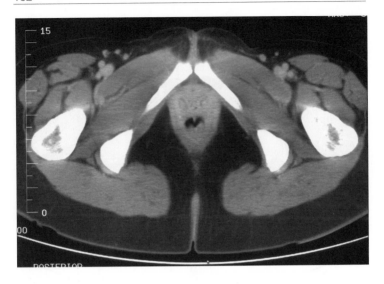

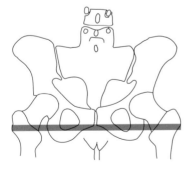

1 Gluteal fascia
2 Vastus lateralis muscle
3 Lateral femoral circumflex artery
4 Iliopsoas muscle
5 Femoral nerve
6 Lateral femoral circumflex artery and vein
7 Obturator artery and vein
8 Superficial epigastric artery and vein
9 Great saphenous vein
10 Pectineus muscle
11 Adductor brevis muscle
12 Bulbocavernosus muscle
13 Vagina
14 Urethra
15 Clitoris
16 Pubic bone (inferior ramus)
17 External obturator muscle
18 Internal obturator muscle
19 Femoral artery and vein

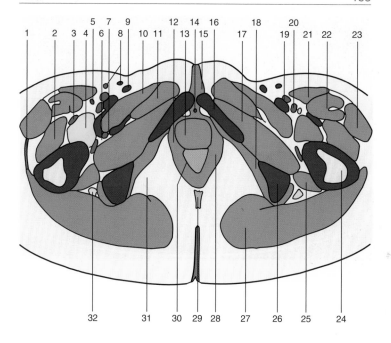

20 Deep femoral artery
21 Sartorius muscle
22 Rectus femoris muscle
23 Tensor fasciae latae muscle
24 Femur
25 Quadratus femoris muscle
26 Ischium
27 Gluteus maximus muscle
28 External anal sphincter
29 Anococcygeal ligament
30 Anal canal
31 Ischiorectal fossa
32 Sciatic nerve
33 Deep inguinal lymph nodes
34 Superficial inguinal lymph nodes
35 Paravaginal lymph nodes
36 Pararectal lymph nodes

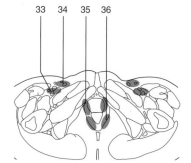

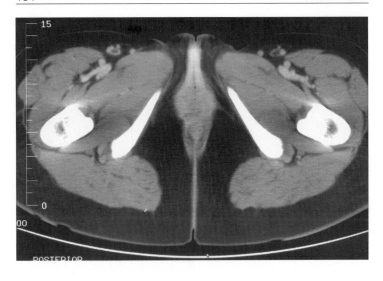

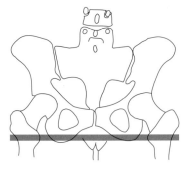

1   Iliopsoas muscle
2   Lateral femoral circumflex artery and vein
3   Deep femoral artery
4   Superficial epigastric artery and vein
5   Adductor longus muscle
6   Adductor magnus muscle
7   Adductor brevis muscle
8   Superficial transverse perineal muscle
9   Bulbocavernosus muscle
10 Clitoris
11 Urethra
12 Bulb of vestibule
13 Gracilis muscle
14 Ischium
15 Great saphenous vein
16 Femoral artery and vein
17 Pectineus muscle
18 Lateral femoral circumflex artery and vein
19 Sartorius muscle

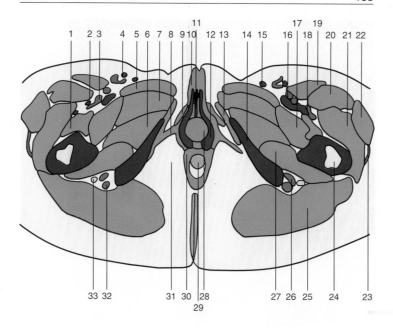

20 Rectus femoris muscle
21 Vastus lateralis muscle
22 Tensor fasciae latae muscle
23 Iliotibial tract
24 Femur
25 Gluteus maximus muscle
26 Semimembranosus muscle (tendon)
27 Quadratus femoris muscle
28 Vagina
29 Anal canal
30 External anal sphincter
31 Ischiorectal fossa
32 Biceps femoris and semitendinosus
   (tendon) muscles
33 Sciatic nerve
34 Deep inguinal lymph nodes
35 Superficial inguinal lymph nodes
36 Paravaginal lymph nodes
37 Anorectal lymph nodes

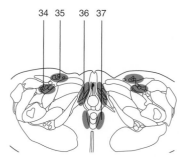

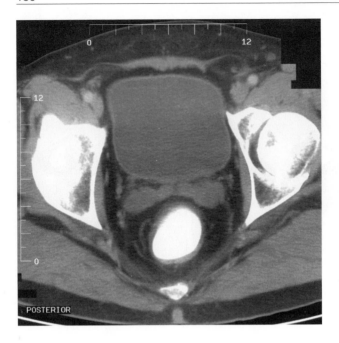

1 Spermatic cord
2 Vas deferens
3 Ureter
4 Ampulla of vas deferens
5 Seminal vesicle
6 Corpus cavernosum
7 Urethra (prostatic part)
8 Suspensory ligament of penis
9 Prostate gland
10 Spermatic artery and vein

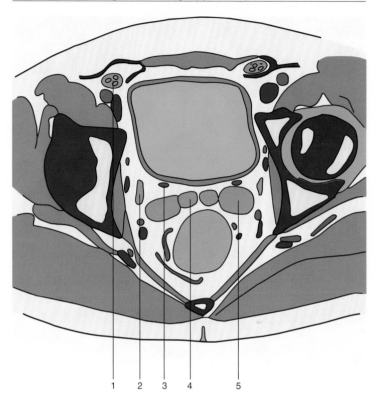

1   2   3   4   5

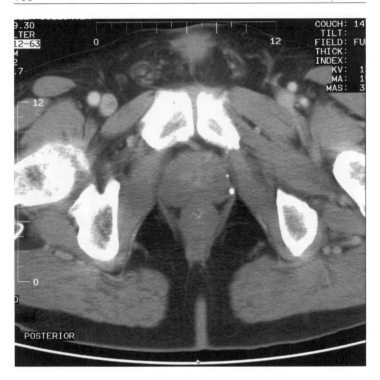

1 Spermatic cord
2 Vas deferens
3 Ureter
4 Ampulla of vas deferens
5 Seminal vesicle
6 Corpus cavernosum
7 Urethra (prostatic part)
8 Suspensory ligament of penis
9 Prostate gland

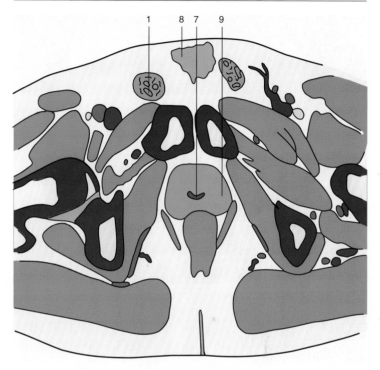

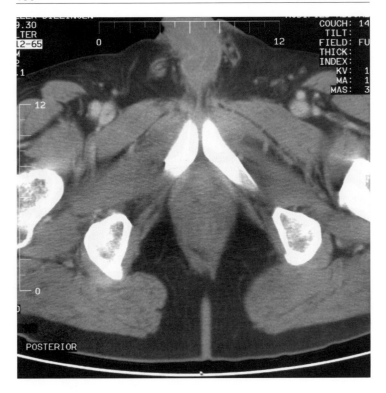

1 Spermatic cord
2 Vas deferens
3 Ureter
4 Ampulla of vas deferens
5 Seminal vesicle
6 Corpus cavernosum
7 Urethra (prostatic part)
8 Suspensory ligament of penis
9 Prostate gland
10 Spermatic artery and vein

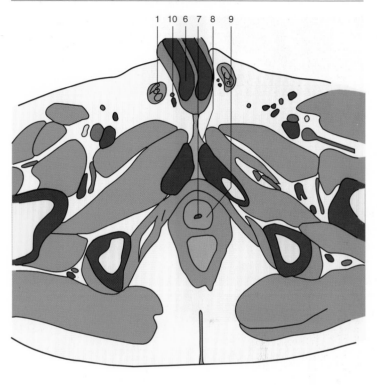

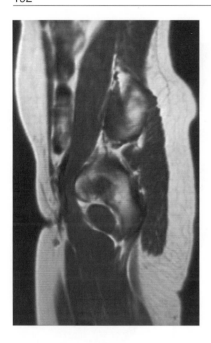

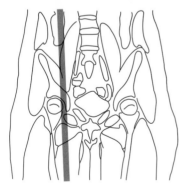

1 Jejunum
2 Psoas muscle
3 Ascending colon
4 Rectus abdominis muscle
5 Superior gluteal artery
6 External iliac artery
7 Pubic bone
8 Pectineus muscle
9 Deep femoral artery
10 Superficial femoral artery
11 Great saphenous vein
12 Adductor brevis muscle
13 Adductor longus muscle
14 Sartorius muscle
15 Longissimus thoracis muscle
16 Quadratus lumborum muscle
17 Lumbar artery
18 Ilium
19 Iliacus muscle
20 Sacrum
21 Gluteus maximus muscle
22 Piriformis muscle
23 Inferior gluteal artery
24 Superior gluteal artery

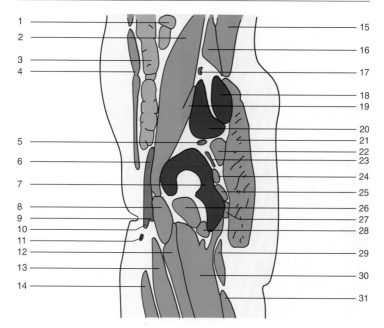

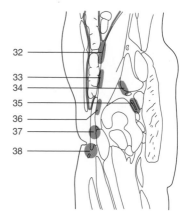

25 Internal obturator muscle
26 External obturator muscle
27 Inferior gluteal artery
28 Quadratus femoris muscle
29 Semitendinosus muscle
30 Adductor longus muscle
31 Semitendinosus muscle
32 Paracolic lymph nodes
33 Lateral external iliac lymph nodes
34 Superior gluteal lymph nodes
35 Inferior gluteal lymph nodes
36 Intermediate external iliac lymph nodes
37 Deep inguinal lymph nodes
38 Superficial inguinal lymph nodes

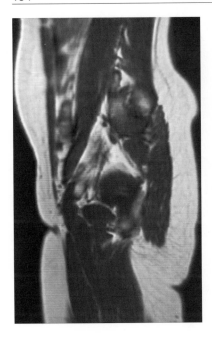

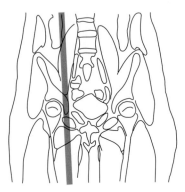

1 Psoas muscle
2 Jejunal artery and vein
3 Jejunum
4 Rectus abdominis muscle
5 External iliac artery
6 Inferior epigastric artery
7 Obturator artery and vein
8 Pubic bone
9 External iliac vein
10 External obturator muscle
11 Pectineus muscle
12 Adductor brevis muscle
13 Adductor longus muscle
14 Longissimus thoracis muscle
15 Ilium
16 Sacrum
17 Internal iliac artery and vein
18 Superior gluteal vein
19 Piriformis muscle
20 Inferior gluteal artery
21 Levator ani muscle
22 Internal pudendal artery
23 Internal obturator muscle
24 Gluteus maximus muscle

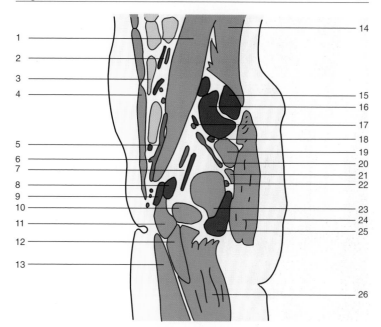

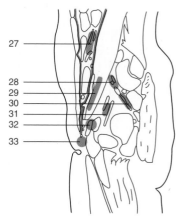

25 Ischial tuberosity
26 Adductor magnus muscle
27 Juxtaintestinal lymph nodes
28 Superior gluteal lymph nodes
29 Intermediate external iliac lymph nodes
30 Inferior gluteal lymph nodes
31 External iliac obturatory lymph nodes
32 Deep inguinal lymph nodes
33 Superficial inguinal lymph nodes

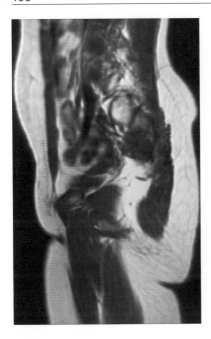

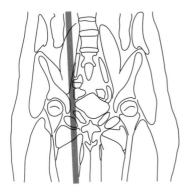

1 Jejunum
2 Ovarian vein
3 Ovarian artery
4 Ureter
5 Common iliac vein
6 External iliac artery
7 Internal iliac artery
8 External iliac vein
9 Rectus abdominis muscle
10 Ileum
11 Pubic bone (superior ramus)
12 Pectineus muscle
13 Adductor brevis muscle
14 Adductor longus muscle
15 Sartorius muscle
16 Spinalis muscle
17 Lumbar vertebra 4
18 Lumbar vein
19 Internal iliac vein
20 Spinal nerve L5
21 Piriformis muscle
22 Sacral plexus
23 Pudendal plexus
24 Ileal artery and vein

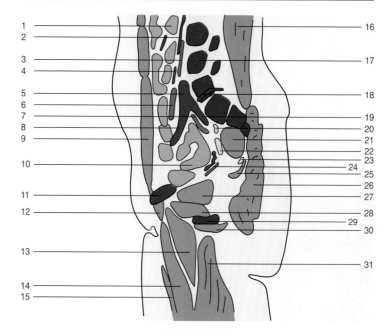

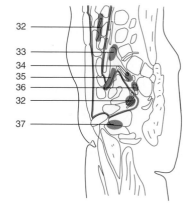

25 Levator ani muscle
26 Gluteus maximus muscle
27 Internal obturator muscle
28 External obturator muscle
29 Pubic bone (inferior ramus)
30 Ischiocavernosus muscle
31 Adductor magnus muscle
32 Juxtaintestinal lymph nodes
33 Medial common iliac lymph nodes
34 Superior gluteal lymph nodes
35 Medial external iliac lymph nodes
36 Inferior gluteal lymph nodes
37 Lateral vesicular lymph nodes

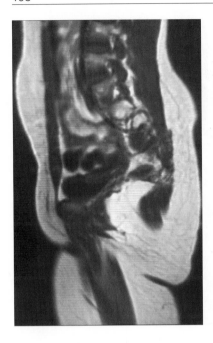

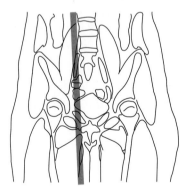

1 Inferior vena cava
2 Jejunum
3 Jejunal artery and vein
4 Right common iliac artery
5 Rectus abdominis muscle
6 Ileum
7 Uterus
8 Urinary bladder
9 Vagina
10 Pubic bone
11 Pectineus muscle
12 Adductor longus muscle
13 Gracilis muscle
14 Adductor magnus muscle
15 Spinalis muscle
16 Lumbar vertebra 5
17 Common iliac vein
18 Median sacral artery
19 Piriformis muscle
20 Rectum
21 Levator ani muscle
22 Gluteus maximus muscle
23 Ischiorectal fossa
24 Ischiocavernosus muscle

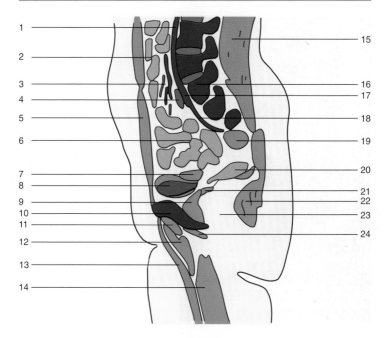

25 Intermediate common iliac lymph nodes
26 Superior gluteal lymph nodes
27 Inferior gluteal lymph nodes
28 Pararectal lymph nodes
29 Postvesicular lymph nodes
30 Prevesicular lymph nodes
31 Paravaginal lymph nodes

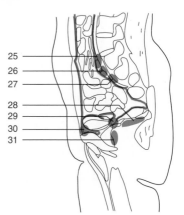

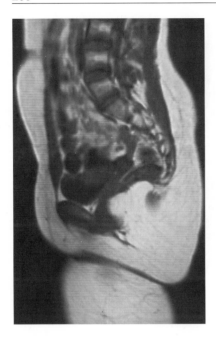

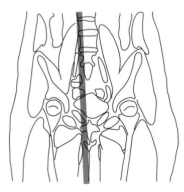

1 Inferior vena cava
2 Umbilicus
3 Right common iliac artery
4 Jejunum
5 Rectus abdominis muscle
6 Ileum
7 Ileal artery and vein
8 Fornix of vagina
9 Uterus
10 Vagina
11 Urinary bladder
12 Pubic bone
13 Pectineus muscle
14 Labium minor
15 Spinal canal
16 Spinalis muscle
17 Lumbar vertebra 5
18 Median sacral artery
19 Rectum
20 Coccyx
21 Levator ani muscle
22 Gluteus maximus muscle
23 Deep transverse perineal muscle
24 Superficial transverse perineal muscle

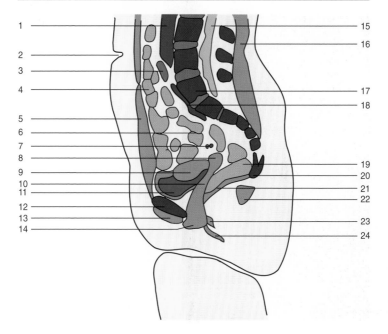

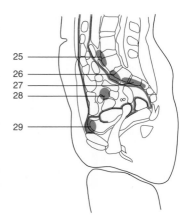

25 Intermediate common iliac lymph nodes
26 Common iliac lymph nodes of promontory
27 Presacral lymph nodes
28 Juxtaintestinal lymph nodes
29 Prevesicular lymph nodes

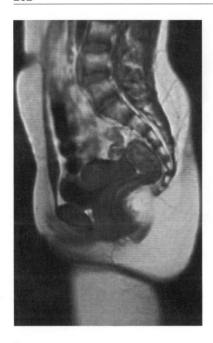

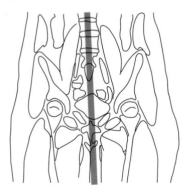

1 Superior mesenteric vein
2 Abdominal aorta
3 Umbilicus
4 Rectus abdominis muscle
5 Jejunal vein
6 Jejunum
7 Ileum
8 Uterus
9 Urinary bladder
10 Urethra
11 Deep perineal space
12 Pubic bone
13 Clitoris
14 Spinalis muscle
15 Left common iliac vein
16 Lumbar vertebra 5
17 Median sacral artery
18 Uterosacral ligament
19 Rectum (ampulla)
20 Rectouterine (Douglas) pouch
21 Coccyx
22 Levator ani muscle
23 Vagina
24 Anal canal

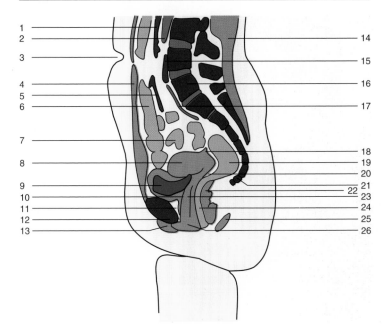

1
2

3

4
5
6

7

8

9
10
11
12
13

14

15

16

17

18
19
20
21
22
23
24
25
26

25 External anal sphincter
26 Labium minor
27 Intermediate common iliac lymph nodes
28 Common iliac lymph nodes of promontory
29 Presacral lymph nodes
30 Juxtaintestinal lymph nodes
31 Prevesicular lymph nodes

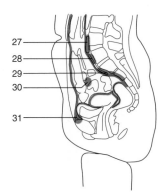

27

28

29

30

31

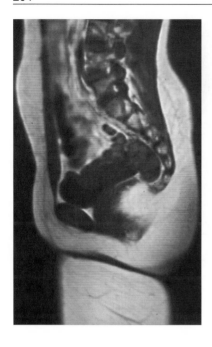

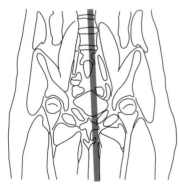

1 Abdominal aorta
2 Jejunum
3 Jejunal artery and vein
4 Rectus abdominis muscle
5 Ileum
6 Uterus
7 Urinary bladder
8 Deep perineal space
9 Pubic bone
10 Spinalis muscle
11 Left common iliac vein
12 Lumbar vertebra 5
13 Ileal artery and vein
14 Rectum (ampulla)
15 Rectouterine (Douglas) pouch
16 Coccyx
17 Vagina
18 Levator ani muscle
19 External anal sphincter
20 Subaortic common iliac lymph nodes
21 Intermediate common iliac lymph nodes
22 Juxtaintestinal lymph nodes
23 Superior gluteal lymph nodes
24 Sacral lymph nodes

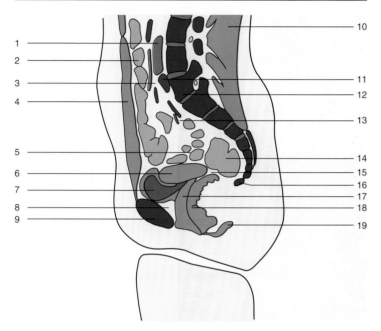

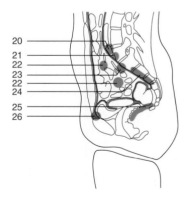

25 Pararectal lymph nodes
26 Prevesicular lymph nodes

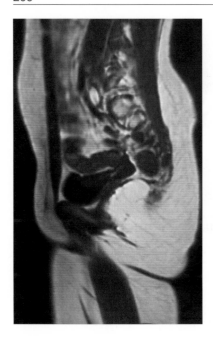

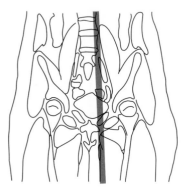

1 Jejunal artery and vein
2 Abdominal aorta
3 Left common iliac vein
4 Jejunum
5 External iliac artery
6 Ileal artery and vein
7 Rectus abdominis muscle
8 Sigmoid colon
9 Uterus
10 Urinary bladder
11 Pubic bone
12 Ischiocavernosus muscle
13 Gracilis muscle
14 Great saphenous vein
15 Psoas muscle
16 Spinalis muscle
17 Sacral vertebra 1
18 Common iliac artery
19 Internal iliac artery
20 Piriformis muscle
21 Rectum
22 Vagina
23 Coccyx
24 Levator ani muscle

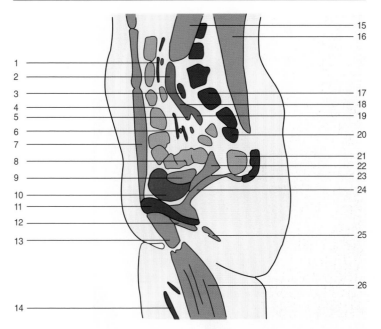

15
16

1
2

3
4
5
6
7

8

9

10
11

12
13

17
18
19

20

21
22
23

24

25

26

14

25 Superficial transverse perineal muscle
26 Adductor longus muscle
27 Juxtaintestinal lymph nodes
28 Intermediate common iliac lymph nodes
29 Superior gluteal lymph nodes
30 Pararectal lymph nodes
31 Paravaginal lymph nodes
32 Prevesicular lymph nodes

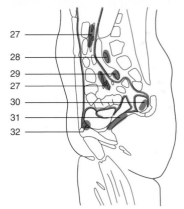

27

28

29
27

30

31

32

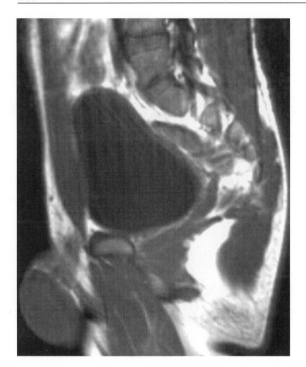

1 Seminal vesicle
2 Spermatic cord
3 Head of epididymis
4 Epididymis
5 Testicle
6 Ampulla of vas deferens
7 Ejaculatory duct
8 Prostate gland
9 Corpus cavernosum
10 Deep dorsal vein of penis
11 Glans penis
12 Urethra (prostate part)
13 Corpus spongiosum
14 Urethra (membranous part)
15 Urogenital diaphragm
16 Urethra (penile or spongy part)

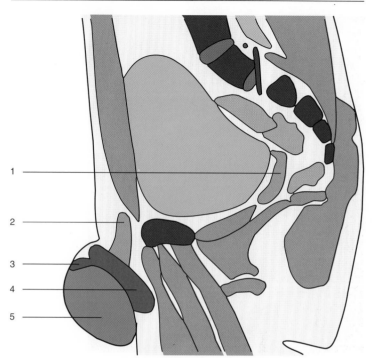

1

2

3

4

5

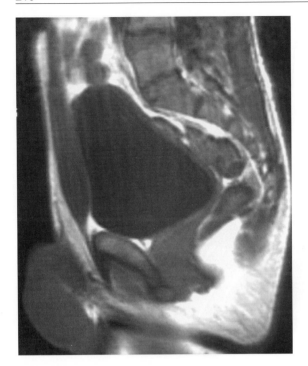

1 Seminal vesicle
2 Spermatic cord
3 Head of epididymis
4 Epididymis
5 Testicle
6 Ampulla of vas deferens
7 Ejaculatory duct
8 Prostate gland
9 Corpus cavernosum
10 Deep dorsal vein of penis
11 Glans penis
12 Urethra (prostate part)
13 Corpus spongiosum
14 Urethra (membranous part)
15 Urogenital diaphragm
16 Urethra (penile or spongy part)

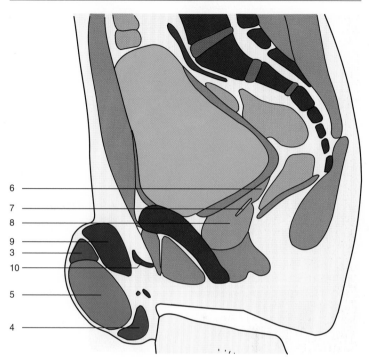

6

7

8

9
3
10

5

4

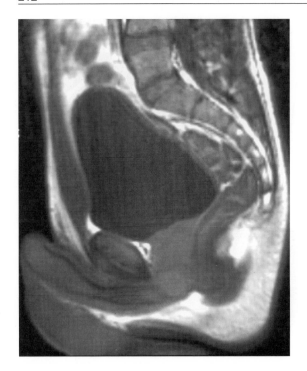

1 Seminal vesicle
2 Spermatic cord
3 Head of epididymis
4 Epididymis
5 Testicle
6 Ampulla of vas deferens
7 Ejaculatory duct
8 Prostate gland
9 Corpus cavernosum
10 Deep dorsal vein of penis
11 Glans penis
12 Urethra (prostate part)
13 Corpus spongiosum
14 Urethra (membranous part)
15 Urogenital diaphragm
16 Urethra (penile or spongy part)

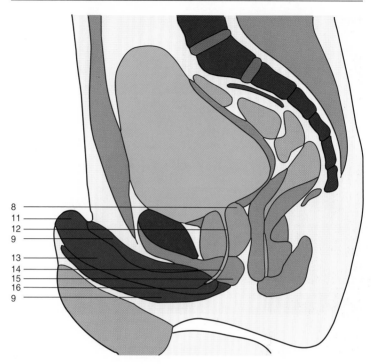

8
11
12
9

13
14
15
16
9

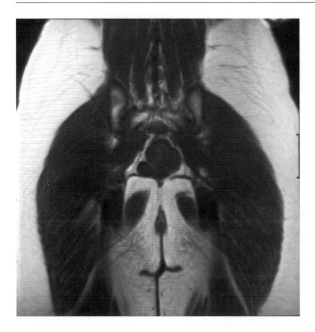

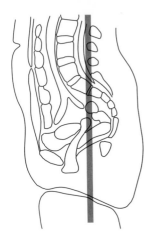

1 Spinalis muscle
2 Longissimus thoracis muscle
3 Iliocostalis lumborum muscle
4 Ilium
5 Sacroiliac joint
6 Sacral plexus
7 Inferior gluteal artery
8 Levator ani muscle
9 Gluteus maximus muscle
10 Biceps femoris muscle
11 Sacrum
12 Piriformis muscle
13 Rectum
14 Uterus
15 Internal pudendal artery
16 Anus
17 Labium major
18 Semitendinosus muscle
19 Common iliac lymph nodes of promontory
20 Superior gluteal lymph nodes
21 Pararectal lymph nodes
22 Pararectal lymph nodes

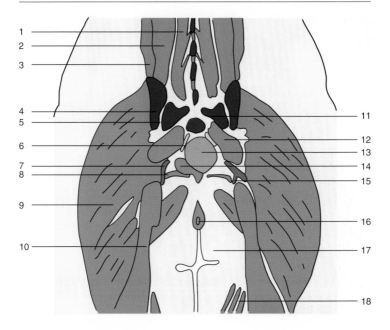

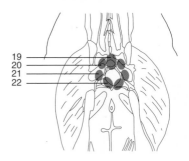

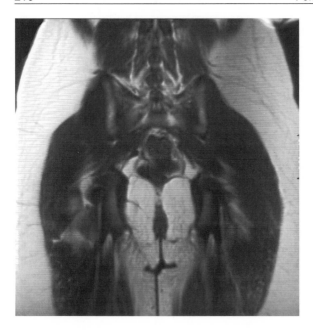

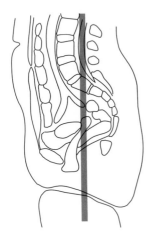

1 Latissimus dorsi muscle
2 Iliocostalis lumborum muscle
3 Longissimus thoracis muscle
4 Spinalis muscle
5 Sacrum
6 Sacroiliac joint
7 Gluteus medius muscle
8 Piriformis muscle
9 Middle rectal artery
10 Uterus
11 External obturator muscle
12 Internal obturator muscle
13 Ischium
14 Greater trochanter
15 Quadratus femoris muscle
16 Labium major
17 Gracilis muscle
18 Gluteus medius muscle
19 Piriformis muscle
20 Superior gluteal artery
21 Rectum
22 Levator ani muscle
23 Inferior gluteal artery
24 Vagina (posterior part)
25 Superficial transverse perineal muscle

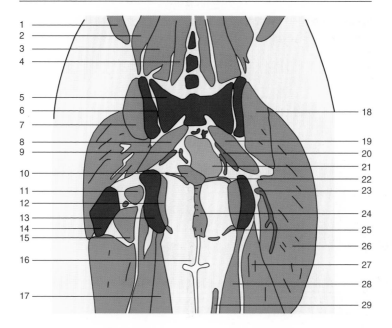

1
2
3
4
5
6
7
8
9
10
11
12
13
14
15
16
17
18
19
20
21
22
23
24
25
26
27
28
29

26 Gluteus maximus muscle
27 Biceps femoris muscle
28 Semitendinosus muscle
29 Gracilis muscle
30 Common iliac lymph nodes of
   promontory
31 Superior gluteal lymph nodes
32 Pararectal lymph nodes
33 Inferior gluteal lymph nodes
34 Parauterine lymph nodes

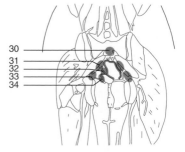

30
31
32
33
34

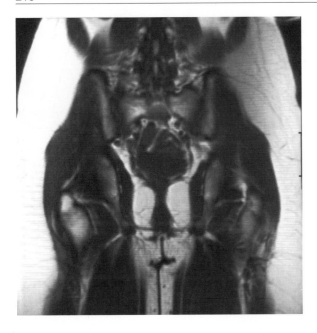

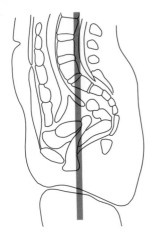

1 Longissimus thoracis muscle
2 External and internal oblique muscles;
   transversus abdominis muscle
3 Ilium (ala)
4 Gluteus medius muscle
5 Superior gluteal artery and vein
6 Uterine artery
7 Gluteus maximus muscle
8 Levator ani muscle
9 Internal obturator muscle
10 Greater trochanter
11 Quadratus femoris muscle
12 Femur
13 Vastus lateralis muscle
14 Adductor magnus muscle
15 Quadratus lumborum muscle
16 Spinalis muscle
17 Internal iliac artery and vein
18 Superior rectal artery and vein
19 Rectum
20 Uterus
21 Cervix (vaginal portion)
22 Internal obturator muscle
23 Ilium
24 Vagina

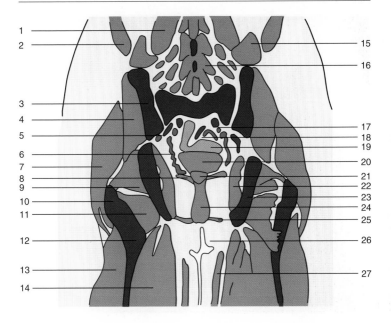

25 Superficial transverse perineal muscle
26 Labium major
27 Gracilis muscle
28 Presacral lymph nodes
29 Superior gluteal lymph nodes
30 Inferior gluteal lymph nodes
31 Parauterine lymph nodes
32 Paravaginal lymph nodes

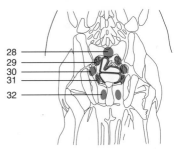

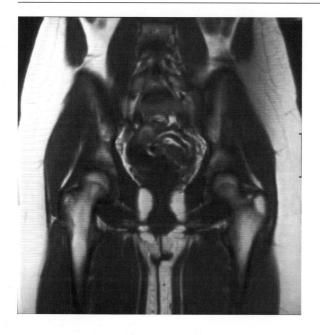

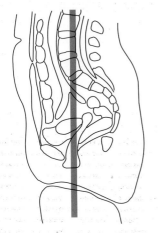

1 External and internal oblique muscles;
   transversus abdominis muscle
2 Psoas muscle
3 Ureter
4 Internal iliac vein
5 Internal iliac artery
6 Ischium (body)
7 Internal obturator muscle
8 Head of femur
9 Uterus
10 Vagina
11 Ischium
12 Adductor brevis muscle
13 Gracilis muscle
14 Adductor magnus muscle
15 Vastus lateralis muscle
16 Iliocostalis lumborum muscle
17 Longissimus thoracis muscle
18 Lumbar vertebra 4
19 Lumbar plexus
20 Sacrum
21 Ilium (ala)
22 Superior rectal artery and vein
23 Rectum
24 Fallopian tube (isthmus)

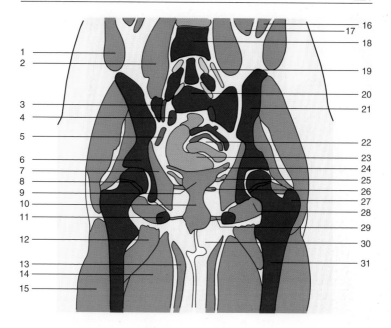

25 Round ligament of uterus
26 Levator ani muscle
27 Greater trochanter
28 External obturator muscle
29 Superficial transverse perineal muscle
30 Labium major
31 Femur
32 Prevertebral lymph nodes
33 Superior gluteal lymph nodes
34 Inferior gluteal lymph nodes
35 Parauterine lymph nodes
36 Paravaginal lymph nodes

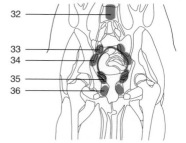

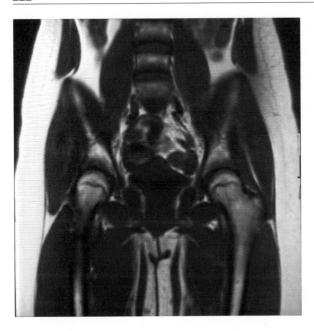

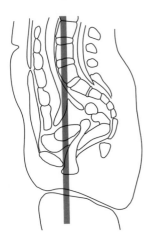

1 Ascending colon
2 External oblique muscle
3 Internal oblique muscle
4 Transversus abdominis muscle
5 Lumbar vertebra 4
6 Iliacus muscle
7 Jejunal vein
8 Ischium
9 Uterus
10 Internal obturator muscle
11 Vagina
12 External obturator muscle
13 Superficial transverse perineal muscle
14 Adductor brevis muscle
15 Jejunum
16 Descending colon
17 Lumbar artery
18 Ilium (ala)
19 Internal iliac artery and vein
20 Gluteus medius muscle
21 Gluteus minimus muscle
22 Ileum
23 Head of femur
24 Greater trochanter
25 Ischium

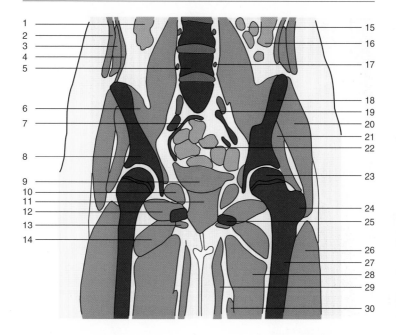

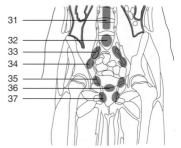

26 Vastus lateralis muscle
27 Femur
28 Adductor magnus muscle
29 Gracilis muscle
30 Sartorius muscle
31 Prevertebral lymph nodes
32 Common iliac lymph nodes of promontory
33 Superior gluteal lymph nodes
34 Inferior gluteal lymph nodes
35 Parauterine lymph nodes
36 Postvesicular lymph nodes
37 Paravaginal lymph nodes

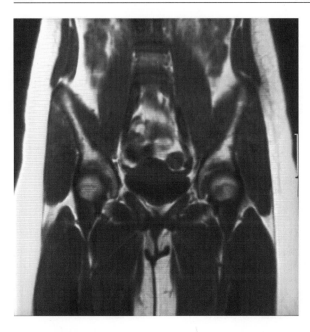

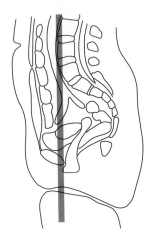

1 Ascending colon
2 External oblique muscle
3 Internal oblique muscle
4 Transversus abdominis muscle
5 Lumbar vertebra 4
6 Psoas muscle
7 Internal iliac artery
8 Iliacus muscle
9 Gluteus medius muscle
10 Gluteus minimus muscle
11 Ureter
12 Head of femur
13 Pubic bone
14 Iliopsoas muscle
15 Tensor fasciae latae muscle
16 Labium major
17 Adductor longus muscle
18 Gracilis muscle
19 Adductor magnus muscle
20 Jejunum
21 Descending colon
22 Ilium
23 Ileum
24 Fallopian tube
25 Uterus

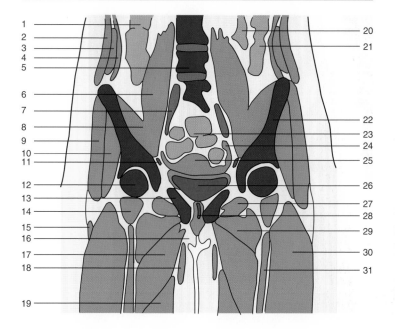

1
2
3
4
5
6
7
8
9
10
11
12
13
14
15
16
17
18
19

20
21
22
23
24
25
26
27
28
29
30
31

26 Urinary bladder
27 External obturator muscle
28 Urethra
29 Adductor brevis muscle
30 Vastus lateralis muscle
31 Vastus intermedius muscle
32 Prevertebral lymph nodes
33 Intermediate common iliac lymph nodes
34 Superior gluteal lymph nodes
35 Parauterine lymph nodes
36 Lateral vesicular lymph nodes

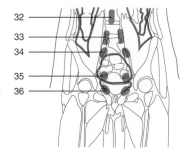

32
33
34
35
36

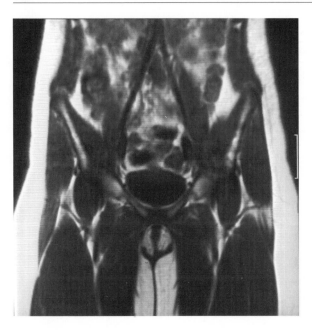

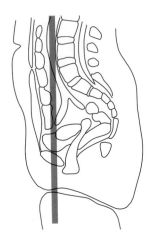

1 Abdominal aorta
2 Ovarian artery and vein
3 Ascending colon
4 Right common iliac artery
5 Psoas muscle
6 Ilium
7 Iliacus muscle
8 Gluteus minimus muscle
9 Gluteus medius muscle
10 Ureter
11 Iliopsoas muscle
12 Lateral femoral circumflex artery
13 Tensor fasciae latae muscle
14 Deep femoral artery
15 Femoral artery
16 Adductor longus muscle
17 Vastus intermedius muscle
18 External oblique muscle
19 Internal oblique muscle
20 Transversus abdominis muscle
21 Ascending colon
22 Jejunal arteries and veins
23 Jejunum
24 External iliac vein
25 Ureter

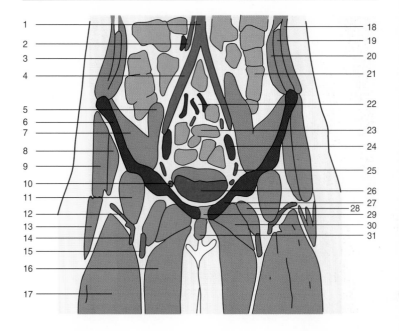

26 Urinary bladder
27 Pubic bone
28 Pectineus muscle
29 Pubic symphysis
30 Adductor brevis muscle
31 Clitoris
32 Subaortic common iliac lymph nodes
33 Lateral common iliac lymph nodes
34 Medial common iliac lymph nodes
35 Lateral external iliac lymph nodes
36 Medial external iliac lymph nodes
37 Superficial inguinal lymph nodes

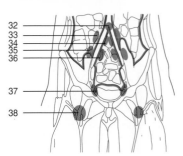

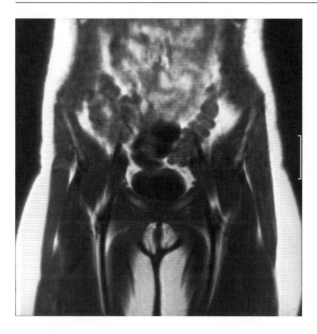

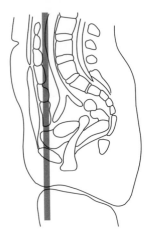

1 Lateral abdominal wall muscle
2 Jejunal arteries and veins
3 Terminal ileum
4 Cecum
5 Sigmoid colon
6 Urinary bladder
7 Pubic symphysis
8 Femoral artery
9 Labium major
10 Femoral vein
11 Great saphenous vein
12 Jejunum
13 Descending colon
14 Ilium
15 Iliacus muscle
16 Tensor fasciae latae muscle
17 External iliac artery
18 Inferior epigastric artery
19 Femoral artery
20 Pubic bone
21 Pectineus muscle
22 Deep femoral artery
23 Clitoris
24 Adductor longus muscle
25 Rectus femoris muscle

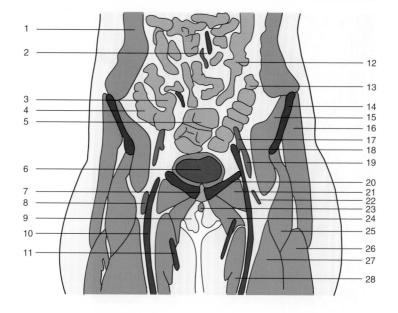

1
2
3
4
5
6
7
8
9
10
11

12
13
14
15
16
17
18
19
20
21
22
23
24
25
26
27
28

26 Vastus lateralis muscle
27 Vastus medialis muscle
28 Sartorius muscle
29 Juxtaintestinal lymph nodes
30 Paracolic lymph nodes
31 Lateral external iliac lymph nodes
32 Medial external iliac lymph nodes
33 Deep inguinal lymph nodes
34 Lateral vesicular lymph nodes
35 Prevesicular lymph nodes
36 Superficial inguinal lymph nodes

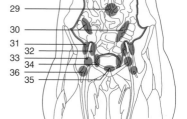

29
30
31
32
33
34
36
35

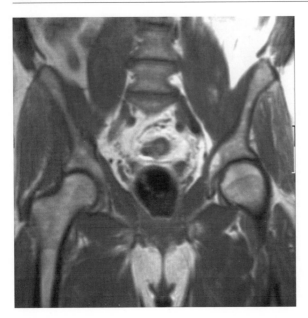

1 Seminal vesicle
2 Ampulla of vas deferens
3 Vas deferens
4 Rectum
5 Prostate gland
6 Urethra (membranous part)
7 Bulbourethral (Cowper s) gland
8 Corpus cavernosum
9 Deep perineal artery
10 Bulb of penis

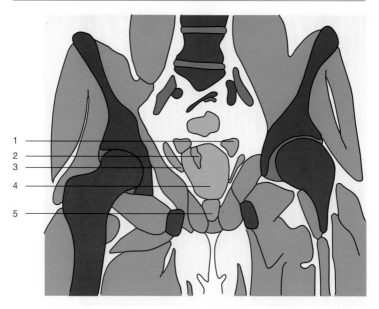

1
2
3
4
5

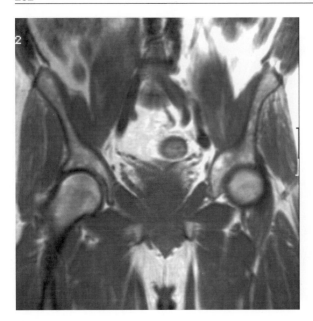

1 Seminal vesicle
2 Ampulla of vas deferens
3 Vas deferens
4 Rectum
5 Prostate gland
6 Urethra (membranous part)
7 Bulbourethral (Cowper's) gland
8 Corpus cavernosum
9 Deep perineal artery
10 Bulb of penis

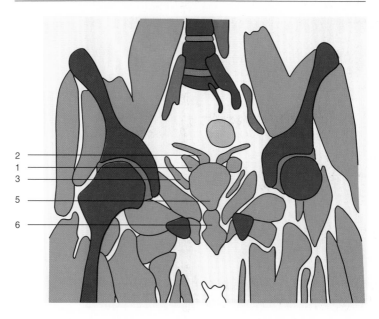

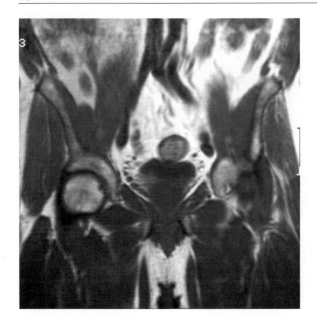

1 Seminal vesicle
2 Ampulla of vas deferens
3 Vas deferens
4 Rectum
5 Prostate gland
6 Urethra (membranous part)
7 Bulbourethral (Cowper's) gland
8 Corpus cavernosum
9 Deep perineal artery
10 Bulb of penis

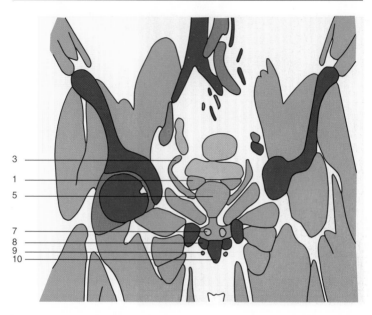

3

1

5

7
8
9
10

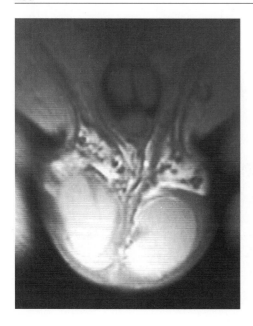

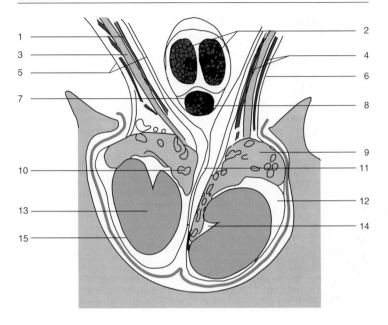

1 Testicular artery
2 Corpus cavernosum
3 Vas deferens
4 Venous plexus
5 Inguinal canal
6 Internal oblique muscle
7 Corpus spongiosum
8 Urethra
9 Head of epididymis
10 Tail of epididymis
11 Septum of scrotum
12 Small hydrocele
13 Testicle
14 Mediastinum testes
15 Tunica albuginea

References

Cahill, D.R., M.J. Orland, C.C. Reading: Atlas of Human Cross-Sectional Anatomy. Wiley-Liss, New York 1990

Chacko A.K., R.W. Katzberg, A. Mac Kay: MRI Atlas of Normal Anatomy. Mc Graw-Hill, New York 1991

El-Khoury G.Y., R.A. Bergmann, W.J. Montgomery: Sectional Anatomy by MRI/CT. Churchill Livingstone, New York 1990

Frick H. Hrsg.: Wolf Heideggers Atlas der Human Anatomie. Karger, Basel 1990

Von Hagens et al.: The Visible Human Body. Lea and Febinger, Philadelphia 1991

Han, Man-Chung, Chu-Wan Kim: Sectional Human Anatomy. Ilchokak, Seoul 1989

Koritke, J.-G., H. Sick: Atlas of Sectional Human Anatomy. Urban & Schwarzenberg, München 1988

Mousavi, S.M., H. Laske, E. Steiner: Atlas der Schnittanatomie und Radiologie. W. Mandrich, Wien 1989

Möller, T.B., E. Reif: Pocket Atlas of Radiographic Anatomy. Thieme, Stuttgart 1992

Richter, E., T. Feyerabend: Normal Lymph Node Topographie. Springer, Berlin 1991

Rohen, I.W.: Anatomie des Menschen. Schattauer, Stuttgart 1988

Witzig, H.: Punkt-Punkt-Komma-Strich, Falken, Niedernhausen 1986

Index